Getting Older

Editor: Danielle Lobban

Volume 464

independence
educational publishers

First published by

Independence Educational Publishers
The Studio, High Green
Great Shelford
Cambridge CB22 5EG
England

www.independence.co.uk

ISBN-13: 978 1 86168 924 5

Printed in Great Britain
Printed and bound by the Pureprint Group using its environmental print technology, a low-carbon, low-waste independently audite process that reduces environmental impact using 100% renewable energy, vegetable-oil-based inks and no industrial alcohol. 98% of a dry waste and 95% of press cleaning solvents are recycled. Pureprint are ISO 14001, EMAS and FSC certified and holds the Queen's Awar for Enterprise: Sustainable Development.

EU Authorised Representative: Easy Access System Europe – Mustamäe tee 50, 10621 Tallinn, Estonia
Web: www.easproject.com Email: gpsr.requests@easproject.com

FSC www.fsc.org MIX Paper | Supporting responsible forestry FSC® C022913

Acknowledgements

The publisher is grateful for permission to reproduce the material in this book. While every care has been taken to trace and acknowledge copyright, the publisher tenders its apology for any accidental infringement or where copyright has proved untraceable. The publisher would be pleased to come to a suitable arrangement in any such case with the rightful owner.

The material reproduced in **issues** books is provided as an educational resource only. The views, opinions and information contained within reprinted material in **issues** books do not necessarily represent those of Independence Educational Publishers and its employees.

Although every effort has been made to ensure that website addresses are correct at time of going to press, Independence Educational Publishers cannot be held responsible for the content of any website mentioned in this book.

Images

Cover image courtesy of Freepik. All other images courtesy of Freepik, Pixabay, Pexels, and Unsplash.

Additional acknowledgements

With thanks to the Independence team: Janey Hills, Klaudi Sommer and Jackie Staines.

Danielle Lobban

Cambridge, September 2025

Contents

Introduction

Getting Older is volume 464 in the **issues** series. The aim of the series is to offer current, diverse information about important issues in our world, from a UK perspective.

About *Getting Older*

With average life expectancy in the UK increasing, more people are living into old age – but what does that really mean? This book explores the emotional, physical, and social challenges elderly people face, helping you to understand ageing with empathy.

Our sources

Titles in the **issues** series are designed to function as educational resource books, providing a balanced overview of a specific subject.

The information in our books is comprised of facts, articles and opinions from many different sources, including:

- Newspaper reports and opinion pieces
- Website factsheets
- Magazine and journal articles
- Statistics and surveys
- Government reports
- Literature from special interest groups.

A note on critical evaluation

Because the information reprinted here is from a number of different sources, readers should bear in mind the origin of the text and whether the source is likely to have a particular bias when presenting information (or when conducting their research). It is hoped that, as you read about the many aspects of the issues explored in this book, you will critically evaluate the information presented.

It is important that you decide whether you are being presented with facts or opinions. Does the writer give a biased or unbiased report? If an opinion is being expressed, do you agree with the writer? Is there potential bias to the 'facts' or statistics behind an article?

Activities

Throughout this book, you will find a selection of assignments and activities designed to help you engage with the articles you have been reading and to explore your own opinions. Some tasks will take longer than others and there is a mixture of design, writing and research-based activities that you can complete alone or in a group.

Further research

At the end of each article we have listed its source and a website that you can visit if you would like to conduct your own research. Please remember to critically evaluate any sources that you consult and consider whether the information you are viewing is accurate and unbiased.

Issues Online

The **issues** series of books is complemented by our onlin resource, Issues Online.

On the Issues Online website you will find a wealth c information, covering over 75 topics, to support the PSH and RSE curriculum.

Why Issues Online?

Researching a topic? Issues Online is the best place to sta for...

Librarians

Issues Online is an essential tool for librarians: feel confider you are signposting safe, reliable, user-friendly onlin resources to students and teaching staff alike. We provid multi-user concurrent access, so no waiting around fc another student to finish with a resource. Issues Online als provides FREE downloadable posters for your shelf/wal table displays.

Teachers

Issues Online is an ideal resource for lesson plannin inspiring lively debate in class, and setting lessons an homework tasks.

Our accessible, engaging content helps deepen student knowledge, promotes critical thinking, and develop independent learning skills.

Issues Online saves precious preparation time. We wad through the wealth of material on the internet to filter th best quality, most relevant and up-to-date information yo need to start exploring a topic.

Our carefully selected, balanced content presents a overview and insight into each topic from a variety c sources and viewpoints.

Students

Issues Online is designed to support your studies in a broa range of topics, particularly social issues relevant to youn people today.

There are thousands of articles, statistics and infograph instantly available to help you with homework, researcl and assignments.

With 24/7 access using the powerful Algolia search systen you can find relevant information quickly, easily and safel anytime from your laptop, tablet or smartphone, in class c at home.

Visit issuesonline.co.uk to find out more!

issues online
resources for schools, colleges & librarie

Chapter 1

What Does It Mean to Get Older?

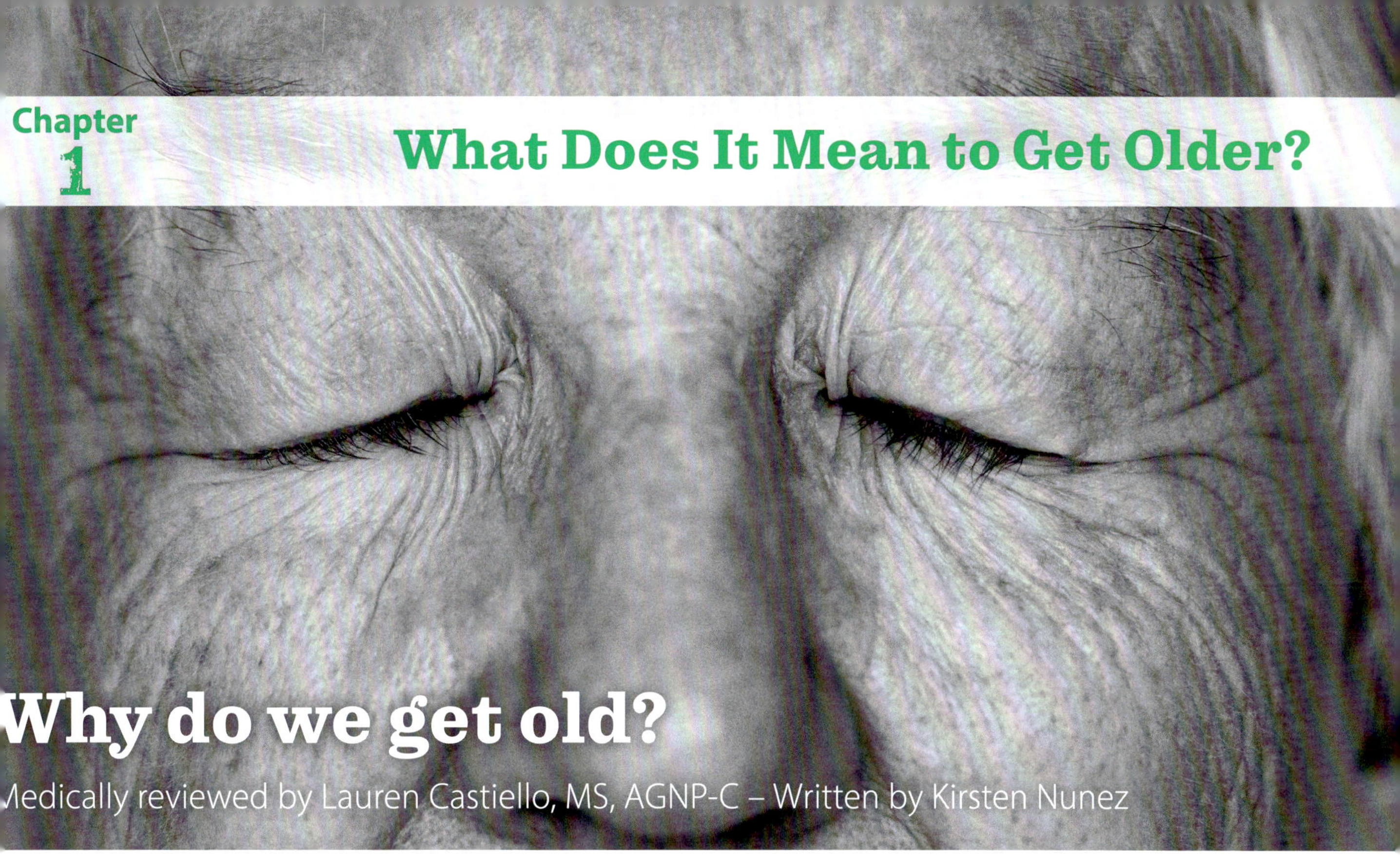

Why do we get old?

ledically reviewed by Lauren Castiello, MS, AGNP-C – Written by Kirsten Nunez

Ageing refers to the physiological changes we experience during our lifespan. It's also an inevitable part of life.

fter all, our cells aren't made to last forever. The structures nd functions in our cells decline over time.

ut why does this happen? For decades, scientists have een studying the subject. There are currently more than 00 theories on why we age, and experts are learning more very day.

et's explore why humans age, and how you can slow down he effects.

Types of ageing

geing can be categorised into two types and due to two ypes of factors, intrinsic and extrinsic.

Intrinsic ageing vs. extrinsic ageing

Intrinsic ageing is a genetically predetermined process that occurs naturally.

Extrinsic ageing is a result of outside factors chosen by you, such as where you live, your stress levels, and your lifestyle habits (like smoking).

ellular ageing

ellular ageing is due to intrinsic factors. It's related to the iological ageing of cells.

ells are the basic building blocks of the body. Your cells re programmed to divide, multiply, and perform basic iological functions.

ut the more cells divide, the older they get. In turn, cells ventually lose their ability to function properly.

ellular damage also increases as cells get older. This makes he cell less healthy, causing biological processes to fail. ellular damage accumulates over time, too.

Damage-related and environmental ageing

Damage-related and environmental ageing is related to extrinsic factors. It refers to how our surroundings and lifestyle affect how we age.

This includes factors like:

- air pollution
- tobacco smoke
- alcohol consumption
- malnutrition
- ultraviolet radiation (UV) exposure

Over time, these factors can damage our cells and contribute to ageing.

Everyone experiences both types of ageing. However, each form of ageing varies from person to person, which explains why we age in different ways.

Theories on ageing

It's generally accepted that ageing is caused by multiple processes, rather than one reason. It's also likely that these processes interact and overlap with each other.

Here are some of the most prominent theories:

Programmed theories of ageing

Programmed ageing theories say that people are designed to age and that our cells have a predetermined lifespan that's encoded into our bodies.

Also called active, or adaptive, ageing theories, they include:

- Gene theory. This theory suggests that specific genes turn 'on' and 'off' over time, causing ageing.
- Endocrine theory. According to this theory, ageing is caused by changes in hormones, which are produced by the endocrine system.

- Immunological theory. Also called the autoimmune theory, this is the idea that the immune response is designed to decline. The result is disease and ageing.

Programmed theories have many supporters. However, they suggest that habits linked to longevity, like quitting smoking and exercise, are useless. This is likely inaccurate, as research has continuously proven that these habits affect life expectancy.

Error theories of ageing

Error theories, or damage theories, are the opposite of programmed theories. They hypothesise that ageing is caused by cellular changes that are random and unplanned.

Error theories of ageing include:

- Wear and tear theory. This is the idea that cells break down and become damaged over time. But critics argue that it doesn't account for the body's ability to repair.
- Genome instability theory. According to this theory, ageing happens because the body loses its ability to repair DNA damage.
- Cross-linkage theory. This theory claims that ageing is due to the buildup of cross-linked proteins, which damages cells and slows biological functions.
- Rate-of-living theory. Proponents of this theory say that an organism's rate of metabolism determines its lifespan. However, the theory lacks solid and consistent scientific evidence.
- Free radical theory. This theory suggests that ageing is due to the buildup of oxidative stress, which is caused by free radicals. But some say this theory fails to explain other types of cellular damage seen in ageing.
- Mitochondrial theory. As a variation of the free radical theory, this theory says that mitochondrial damage releases free radicals and causes ageing. The theory lacks hard scientific evidence.

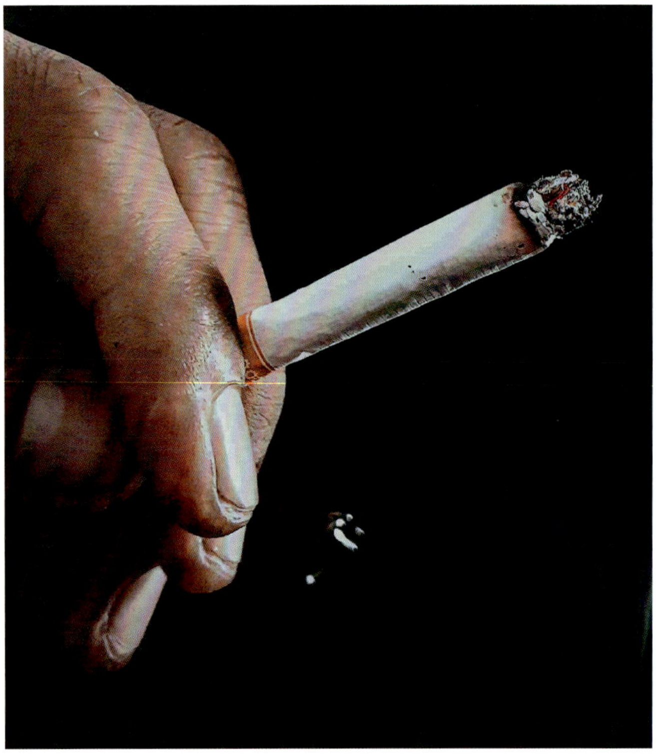

Genetic theory of ageing

The genetic theory proposes that ageing primarily depend on genetics. In other words, our life expectancy is regulate by the genes we got from our parents.

Since genes have predetermined traits, it's thought thi theory overlaps with programmed theories of ageing.

Genetic theories include:

- Telomere theory. Telomeres protect the ends of you chromosomes as they multiply. Over time, telomere shorten, which is associated with disease and ageing.
- Programmed senescence theory. Cellular senescenc occurs when cells stop dividing and growing, but don die. This theory suggests that this causes ageing.
- Stem cell theory. Stem cells can turn into other cell which helps repair tissue and organs. But the functio of stem cells declines over time, potentially contributin to ageing.
- Longevity gene theory. This is the idea that certai genes extend lifespan. More research is necessary.

The limitation of genetic theories is that they disregard th importance of external factors. In fact, it's estimated tha just 25% of lifespan is influenced by genetics. This suggest that environmental and lifestyle factors play a major role.

Evolutionary theory of ageing

Natural selection refers to the adaptive traits of a organism. These traits can help the organism adjust to thei environment, so they're more likely to survive.

According to evolutionary theories, ageing is based o natural selection. It says that an organism begins agein after they have reached their peak of reproduction and hav passed down adaptive traits.

Evolutionary theories include:

- Mutation accumulation. This theory presumes tha random mutations accumulate later in life.
- Antagonistic pleiotropy. According to this theory, gene that promote fertility early in life have negative effect later on.
- Disposable soma theory. The theory claims tha when more metabolic resources are directed towar reproduction, the less is put toward DNA repair. Th result is cell damage and ageing.

These theories are still being researched and require mor evidence.

Biochemical theory of ageing

Another theory is that biochemical reactions caus ageing. These reactions occur naturally and continuousl throughout life.

This theory is rooted in various concepts, including:

- Advanced glycation end products (AGEs). AGEs develo when fats or protein are exposed to sugar. High level may lead to oxidative stress, which speeds up ageing.
- Heat shock response. Heat shock proteins protect cell from stress, but their response decreases as we age.

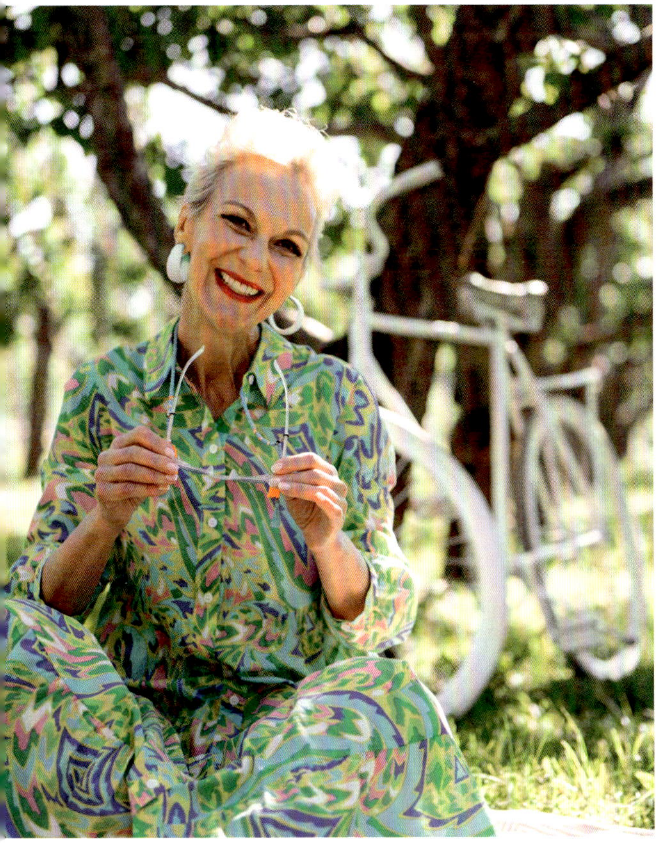

- Damage accumulation. Normal chemical reactions damage DNA, proteins, and metabolites over time.

Why do life expectancies increase?

In recent decades, life expectancy around the world has increased. This is due many factors, including:

- better nutrition
- improved hygiene
- access to healthcare
- improvements in modern medicine

These factors can protect our cells and reduce cellular damage, increasing life expectancy.

Why do women live longer than men?

In most parts of the world, women live longer than men. This is due to several biological, social, and environmental factors.

Women, on average, have more estrogen than men. Estrogen is the female sex hormone. It's been found to have anti-inflammatory and immune-boosting effects, which may protect women from certain diseases.

In contrast, the male sex hormone testosterone may suppress the immune system. Men typically have more of this hormone.

There are also behavioural differences between men and women. Generally, compared to men, women:

- eat healthier
- drive more safely
- consume less alcohol, tobacco, or drugs
- are more likely to access health services

Can we slow the effects of ageing?

Though ageing is inevitable, it's possible to slow down some of the effects. You can do this by following healthy lifestyle habits.

Here's how to slow ageing:

- Eat a nutritious diet. Focus on fruits, vegetables, whole grains, and lean protein. Limit processed foods.
- Stay active. Exercise reduces the physical and mental effects of ageing. Aim for 30 minutes a day, 5 days a week.
- Avoid tobacco. Tobacco speeds up ageing. Quitting is often difficult, but a doctor can help create a cessation plan that works for you.
- Drink alcohol in moderation. Alcohol increases your risk of chronic disease.
- Attend regular checkups. Routine checkups with a doctor are the best way to prevent or treat disease early.
- Know your family history. Discuss your family's health history with your doctor to have appropriate screening or get early treatment for potential chronic diseases.
- Engage your brain. Protect your cognitive function by doing brain exercises.
- Wear sunscreen. Sunscreen protects your skin from UV radiation, which can lead to premature ageing.

Takeaway

Ageing is likely caused by a combination of reasons. Some theories suggest cells have a predetermined lifespan, while others claim it's caused by error and damage. Other theories say that ageing is due to genetic, evolution, or biochemical reactions.

Ageing is normal, but following a healthy lifestyle may help you live longer. Habits like eating well, exercising regularly, and wearing sunscreen can reduce your risk of disease and improve your quality of life.

23 March 2021

www.healthline.com

Understanding theories of ageing activity

In small groups, talk about the different theories of ageing mentioned in the article.

Share your thoughts on which theory you think best explains why we age.

Do you believe that one theory is more accurate than the others, or do you think ageing is caused by a mix of different factors?

Be ready to share a summary of your group's ideas with the class.

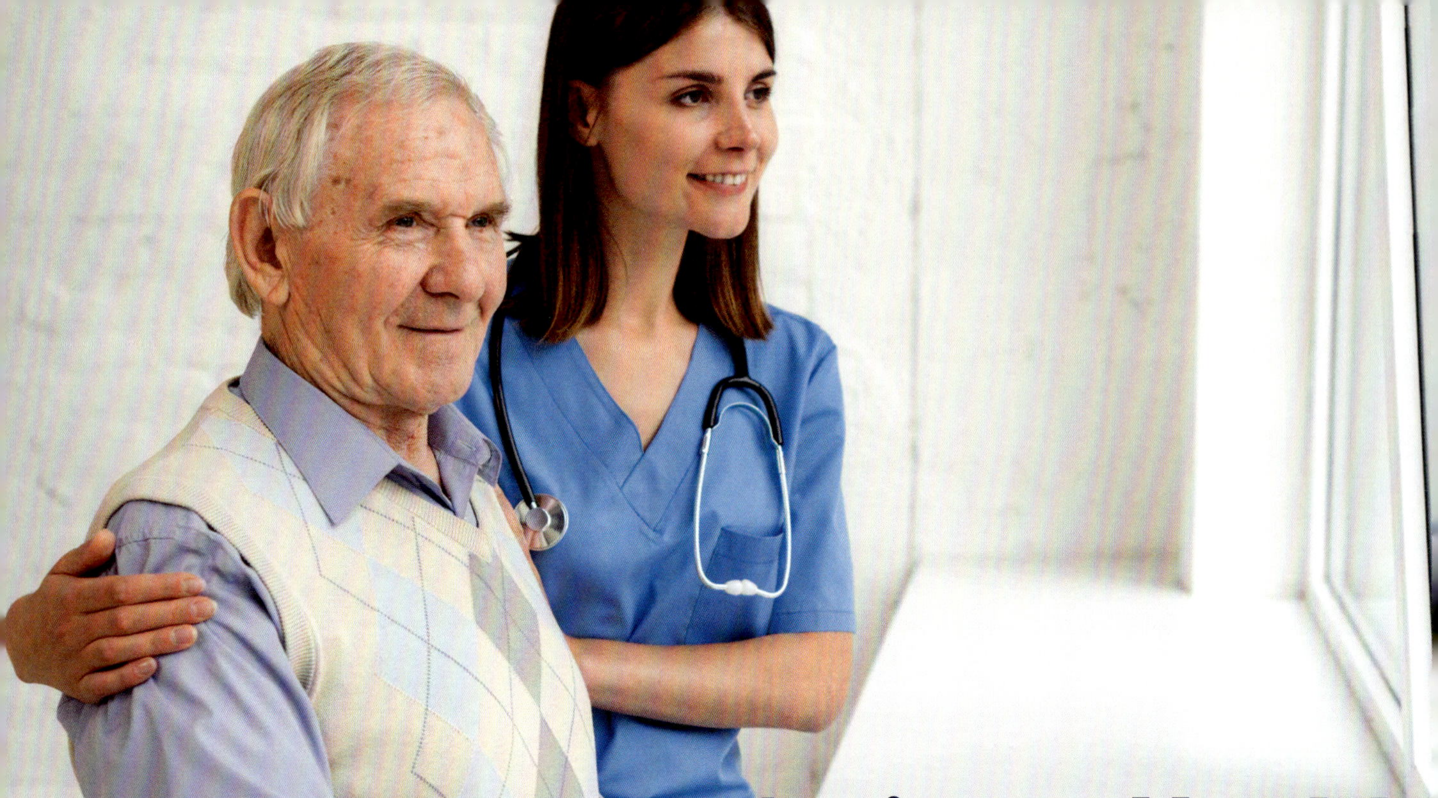

Ageing and health

Key facts

- All countries face major challenges to ensure that their health and social systems are ready to make the most of this demographic shift.
- In 2050, 80% of older people will be living in low- and middle-income countries.
- The pace of population ageing is much faster than in the past.
- In 2020, the number of people aged 60 years and older outnumbered children younger than 5 years.
- Between 2015 and 2050, the proportion of the world's population over 60 years will nearly double from 12% to 22%.

People worldwide are living longer. Today most people can expect to live into their sixties and beyond. Every country in the world is experiencing growth in both the size and the proportion of older persons in the population.

By 2030, one in six people in the world will be aged 60 years or over. At this time the share of the population aged 60 years and over will increase from 1 billion in 2020 to 1.4 billion. By 2050, the world's population of people aged 60 years and older will double (2.1 billion). The number of persons aged 80 years or older is expected to triple between 2020 and 2050 to reach 426 million.

While this shift in distribution of a country's population towards older ages – known as population ageing – started in high-income countries (for example, in Japan 30% of the population is already over 60 years old), it is now low- and middle-income countries that are experiencing the greatest change. By 2050, two-thirds of the world's population over 60 years will live in low- and middle-income countries.

Ageing explained

At the biological level, ageing results from the impact of the accumulation of a wide variety of molecular and cellular damage over time. This leads to a gradual decrease in physical and mental capacity, a growing risk of disease and ultimately death. These changes are neither linear nor consistent, and they are only loosely associated with a person's age in years. The diversity seen in older age is not random. Beyond biological changes, ageing is often associated with other life transitions such as retirement, relocation to more appropriate housing and the death of friends and partners.

Common health conditions associated with ageing

Common conditions in older age include hearing loss, cataracts and refractive errors, back and neck pain and osteoarthritis, chronic obstructive pulmonary disease, diabetes, depression and dementia. As people age, they are more likely to experience several conditions at the same time.

Older age is also characterised by the emergence of several complex health states commonly called geriatric syndromes. They are often the consequence of multiple underlying factors and include frailty, urinary incontinence, falls, delirium and pressure ulcers.

Factors influencing healthy ageing

A longer life brings with it opportunities, not only for older people and their families, but also for societies as a whole.

dditional years provide the chance to pursue new activities ıch as further education, a new career or a long-neglected assion. Older people also contribute in many ways to ıeir families and communities. Yet the extent of these pportunities and contributions depends heavily on one ıctor: health.

vidence suggests that the proportion of life in good health as remained broadly constant, implying that the additional ears are in poor health. If people can experience these extra ears of life in good health and if they live in a supportive nvironment, their ability to do the things they value will be ttle different from that of a younger person. If these added ears are dominated by declines in physical and mental apacity, the implications for older people and for society re more negative.

lthough some of the variations in older people's health re genetic, most is due to people's physical and social nvironments – including their homes, neighbourhoods, nd communities, as well as their personal characteristics such as their sex, ethnicity, or socioeconomic status. he environments that people live in as children – or even s developing foetuses – combined with their personal haracteristics, have long-term effects on how they age.

hysical and social environments can affect health directly r through barriers or incentives that affect opportunities, ecisions and health behaviour. Maintaining healthy ehaviours throughout life, particularly eating a balanced liet, engaging in regular physical activity and refraining from tobacco use, all contribute to reducing the risk of non-communicable diseases, improving physical and mental capacity and delaying care dependency.

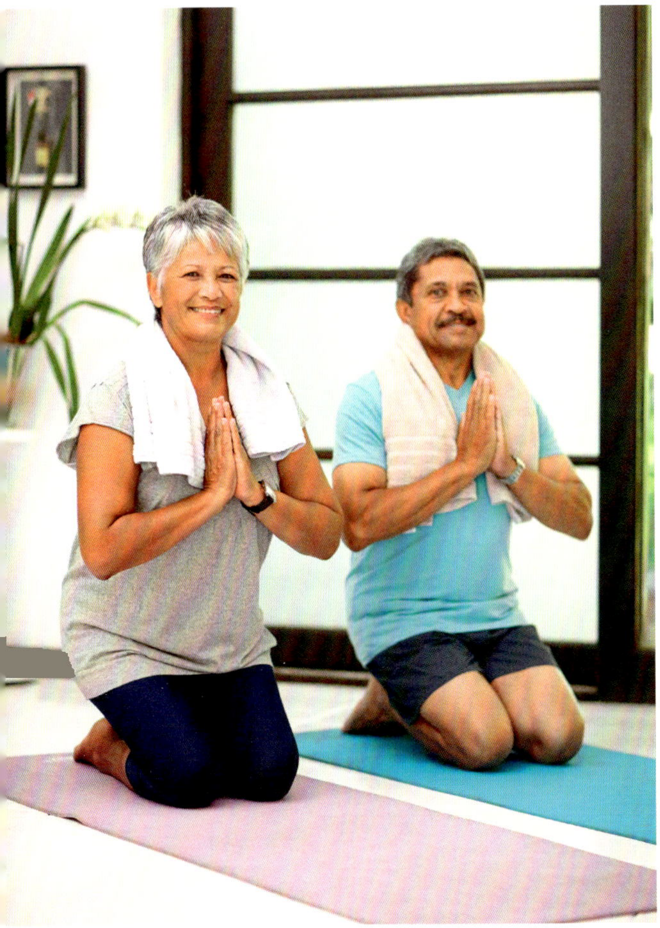

Supportive physical and social environments also enable people to do what is important to them, despite losses in capacity. The availability of safe and accessible public buildings and transport, and places that are easy to walk around, are examples of supportive environments. In developing a public-health response to ageing, it is important not just to consider individual and environmental approaches that ameliorate the losses associated with older age, but also those that may reinforce recovery, adaptation and psychosocial growth.

Challenges in responding to population ageing

There is no typical older person. Some 80-year-olds have physical and mental capacities similar to many 30-year-olds. Other people experience significant declines in capacities at much younger ages. A comprehensive public health response must address this wide range of older people's experiences and needs.

The diversity seen in older age is not random. A large part arises from people's physical and social environments and the impact of these environments on their opportunities and health behaviour. The relationship we have with our environments is skewed by personal characteristics such as the family we were born into, our sex and our ethnicity, leading to inequalities in health.

Older people are often assumed to be frail or dependent and a burden to society. Public health professionals, and society as a whole, need to address these and other ageist attitudes, which can lead to discrimination, affect the way policies are developed and the opportunities older people have to experience healthy ageing.

Globalisation, technological developments (e.g., in transport and communication), urbanisation, migration and changing gender norms are influencing the lives of older people in direct and indirect ways. A public health response must take stock of these current and projected trends and frame policies accordingly.

1 October 2024

www.who.int

Fear of ageing is really a fear of the unknown – and modern society is making thing worse

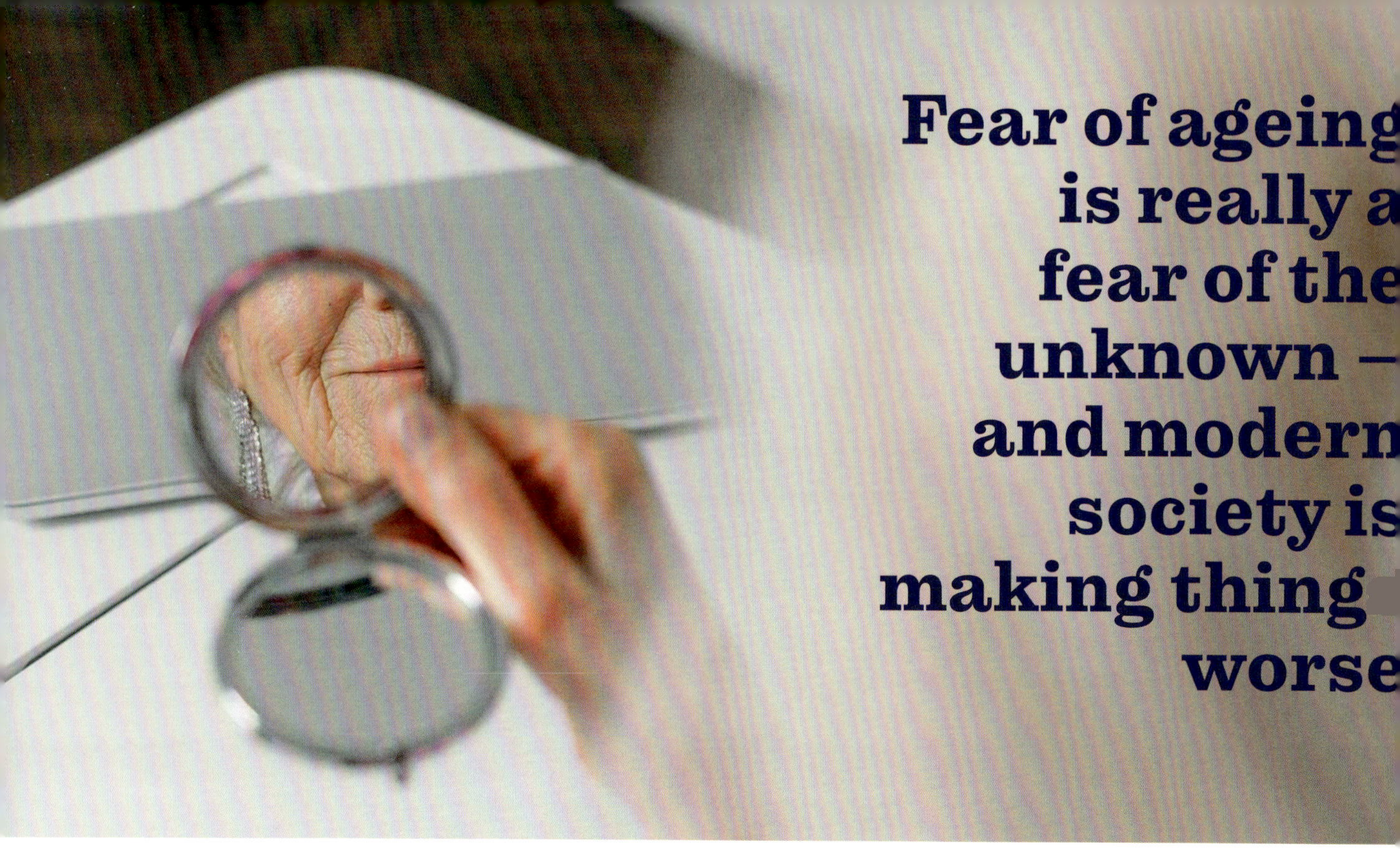

An article from The Conversation.

By Chao Fang, Lecturer in Sociology, Deputy Director of the Centre for Ageing and the Life Course, University of Liverpool and Alastair Comery, PhD Candidate, Sociology, Centre fo Death and Society, University of Bath

For the first time in human history, we have entered an era in which reaching old age is taken for granted. Unlike in ages past, when living to an older age was a luxury afforded mainly to the privileged, globally around 79% of women and 70% of men can expect to reach the age of 65 and beyond.

Despite longer life expectancy, many people in the contemporary west see growing old as undesirable and even scary. Research shows, however, that anxiety about ageing may in fact be fear of the unknown.

Society's focus on youthfulness and capability can cause anxiety about becoming weak and unwanted. Adverts for anti-ageing products are everywhere, reinforcing the idea that growing older is inherently unattractive.

Some people fear ageing so much that it becomes a pathological condition called gerascophobia, leading to irrational thoughts and behaviour, for example, a fixation on health, illness and mortality and a preoccupation with hiding the signs of ageing.

We frequently hear about attempts to reverse ageing, often by the super rich. For example, Bryan Johnson, a 45-year-old American entrepreneur, is spending millions of dollars a year to obtain the physical age of 18.

While the desire to reverse ageing is not a new phenomenon, advancements in biomedicine have brought it closer.

Work published by genetics professor David Sinclair a Harvard University in 2019 suggests that it may be possible to challenge the limits of cell reproduction to extend ou lifespan, for example. His information theory of ageing argues that reprogramming DNA can improve damaged and old tissues, and delay or even reverse ageing. However these new possibilities can also heighten our fear of ageing

From the unproductive to undervalued

People haven't always dreaded growing older. In many societies, older people used to be widely regarded as wise and important – and in some they still are.

In ancient China, there was a culture of respecting and seeking advice from older family members. There is still an ethos of filial piety (showing reverence and care for elders and ancestors) today, even if it's not as pronounced as it used to be. The same went for medieval Europe, where older people's experiences and wisdom were highly valued.

However, the industrial revolution in the west from the 18th century led to a cultural shift where older people became excluded from society and were considered unproductive People who had surpassed the age to work, alongside those with incurable diseases, were regarded by society as 'evils' in need of assistance.

The treatment of older people has taken a different form since the early 20th century. The introduction of universal pension systems made ageing a central concern in welfare systems. But as the demands for social and health care have increased, journalists increasingly portray ageing as a burden on society.

Consequently, growing older is often associated with managing the risk of ill health and alleviating the onus of care from younger relatives. This can result in the institutionalisation of older people in residential facilities that keep them hidden, sequestered from the awareness of younger generations.

Research analysing the responses of 1,200 US adults from the American Association of Retired Persons' Images of Ageing survey shows that much of the perceived fear of ageing is closely aligned with the fear of the unknown, rather than the ageing process itself. This fear is only exacerbated by the largely separate lives lived by older and younger generations.

The prevalence of nuclear families and the decline of traditional mixed-generational communities have deprived younger people of the opportunity to more fully understand the experiences of older people. Plus, the rapid increase in house prices means many young people cannot afford to live near their older relatives.

The separation of older people from children and young people has sparked generational conflicts that seemingly continue to grow wider than ever. Older people are frequently portrayed in the media as conservative and privileged, making it difficult for younger generations to comprehend why older people act and think the way they do.

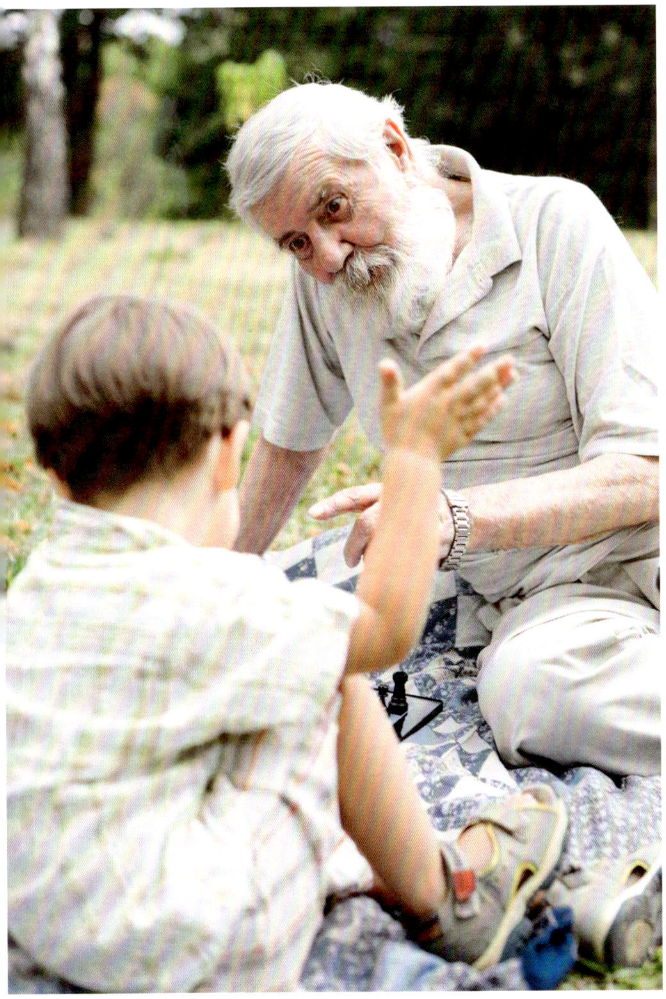

Intergenerational interactions

Academics suggest that creating a system for older and younger generations to interact in everyday settings is vital.

A set of three UK-based studies in 2016 analysed and compared the effects of direct contact, extended contact and interactions between younger (aged 17 to 30) and older people (65 and over). The findings indicated that good quality direct intergenerational contact can improve young people's attitudes towards older adults (especially when sustained over time).

Studies show that these activities can not only enhance the wellbeing of older people but also help younger people gain an appreciation of ageing as a valuable and fulfilling life stage.

Getting worried about growing older is normal, just as we experience anxieties in other stages of life, such as adolescence and marriage. But here's the thing – instead of seeing ageing as a looming figure, it is important to realise it is just a part of life.

Once we understand ageing as a regular experience, we can let go of these worries and approach the journey through different life stages with a positive attitude and a fortified will to enrich our lives and the lives of those around us.

31 January 2024

THE CONVERSATION

The above information is reprinted with kind permission from The Conversation.

www.theconversation.com

What do you imagine ageing will be like?

Write down or draw your first thoughts when you hear the word 'ageing'.

Think about these questions as you do this:

- What do you imagine your life will be like when you are older?
- What worries or excites you about getting older?
- Do you think ageing is scary?

Spend about 5 minutes on this.

Be ready to share your ideas with the class if you want to.

New survey reveals half of people don't believe they will look good when they are old

The new data also reveals that significant proportions of the population have concerns abou their mobility, mental function, competency in their jobs, and ability to drive as they get olde

New Age Without Limits campaign aims to change the way we all think about ageing and support a growing movement working to make society more age-inclusive.

Half of the nation's population (49%) don't think they will look good when they are old, a survey from the newly-launched Age Without Limits anti-ageism campaign reveals.

One in seven (15%) questioned said they don't think they will look good when they are older and are worried about it – rising to one in five (20%) of those surveyed between 30 and 50 years of age.

The Centre for Ageing Better has launched the Age Without Limits campaign this month to tackle the widespread ageism in society which contributes to these overly negative impressions of older age many people hold.

The new research is further indication of how negative stereotypes and misconceptions about ageing shown by the media, the language used in everyday conversation and societal attitudes help fuel negative perceptions of how individuals view their own futures as an older person.

The new Age Without Limits campaign is warning that the internalising of these negative views creates a self-fulfilling prophecy which impacts individual's self-esteem, limits the activities they do and even the clothes they wear.

The three-year campaign will aim to challenge ageism and help change negative attitudes about age and ageing.

The new national survey, which will help track public attitudes towards ageing as the campaign progresses, also reveals that:

- One in two people (46%) don't think they'll be as effective in their job when they are old.
- Almost one in two people (42%) don't think they'll be as good at driving.
- More than a third (38%) of people expect not to have a good social life.
- More than a third (36%) don't think they'll be able to adapt to new technology.

Dr Carole Easton OBE, Chief Executive at the Centre for Ageing Better, said:

'Evidence shows ageism can have a hugely damaging impact on us as we get older not only on how we think about and act towards other people but also on how we view our own ageing.

'If you consider that the public on average considers 58–60 to be old, it is shocking to think that such large proportions of the public don't think they will have good mental functio by this age, or will be able to drive a car as well or be a competent in their jobs.

'Among the most common incorrect assumptions arounc ageing is that it is predominantly about frailty, decline anc dependency. In reality, the large majority of us will not ge dementia or live in care homes, while just one in ten peopl aged 65 are defined as frail.

'Hearing constant negative messaging about older age car become a self-fulfilling prophecy, affecting our self-esteen and what we think we are capable or worthy of as we ge older.

'Thinking negatively about ageing and older people ha been accepted and ignored for too long. Now is the time tc change this. Our new Age Without Limits campaign aims tc spark a national conversation about what ageism is and tc change the way we all think about ageing.'

The survey also shows that the assumed decline in their owr older age is a cause of concern for many with:

- Over a quarter of people (27%) are worried they won't be very mobile when they are old.
- Almost a third (30%) are worried they won't be in gooc physical health.
- More than one in five (21%) are worried they won't have good mental function.
- Around a quarter of people (24%) are worried they won't be independent and will have to rely on others for help.

Analysis of the survey data reveals that younger men (18–29) are more likely than women in their age group to be worried about not looking good, or having poor mobility or having poor mental function as they get older.

But in older age groups, women then become much more likely to worry about the negative expectations of later life.

For example, women aged between 51 and 70 are more than twice as likely to be worried about not looking good when they are older compared to their male counterparts, while women 71 and above are four times more likely to have those concerns than men of the same age.

23 January 2024

www.ageing-better.org.uk

Chapter 2

Inside The Ageing Mind

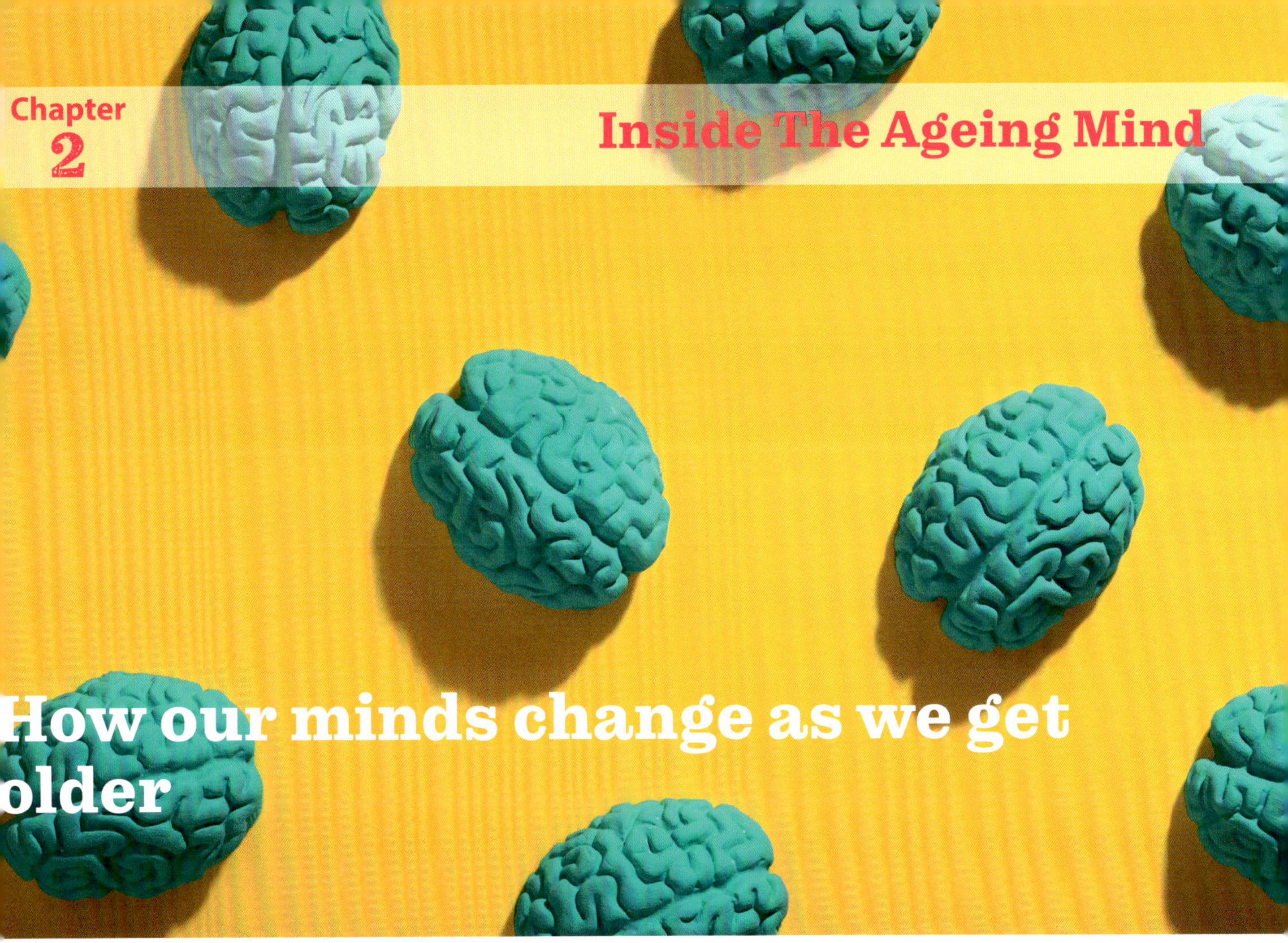

How our minds change as we get older

Getting older is something everyone goes through, and it brings changes to our bodies and minds. It's normal for our thinking and memory to change a bit as we age, but these changes are different for each person. Some people might notice small differences in how quickly they think or remember things, while others stay sharp for a long time. You may have noticed changes in the way your grandparents or other older relatives act, or how they are more forgetful. My grandmother used to say that her mind was so full of memories that she was like a computer running out of storage, some things would have to be deleted to make space for new things!

What changes in thinking are normal?

As people get older, their brains work a little slower. It might take longer to think through problems or react to things around them. Memory can also change, especially when it comes to remembering things for a short time, like a phone number. Paying attention to lots of things at once can be harder too. Sometimes solving problems might take a bit more time, but older people often use their experience and knowledge to help out. These changes are normal and don't mean something is wrong with the brain.

What's happening in the brain?

Inside the brain, some parts get smaller as we age, especially areas important for memory and planning. The connections between brain cells don't work as fast, and the brain isn't as flexible as it used to be, so learning new things can be tougher. However, remembering things learned a long time ago usually stays easier, such as how to tie your shoelaces or ride a bike. The ability to remember things such as phone numbers, passwords and where you parked the car also declines with age.

What affects how our brains age?

How our brains change depends on a lot of things. Staying active by exercising, doing puzzles or games, and hanging out with friends helps keep the brain healthy. Health problems like heart disease or diabetes can make thinking harder, so taking care of your health is important. Your family history also matters, if dementia runs in your family, your risk might be higher. But living a healthy lifestyle can slow down brain changes and help you stay sharp.

Final thoughts

It's normal for thinking and memory to change a little as we get older, but this doesn't mean we will lose all our mental abilities. By staying active, learning new things, and staying social, we can keep our brains strong. Growing older is a chance to keep learning and enjoying life in new ways.

What is dementia?

Dementia is an umbrella term for a range of progressive conditions that affect the brain.

Each type of dementia stops a person's brain cells (neurones) working properly in specific areas, affecting their ability to remember, think and speak.

Doctors typically use the word 'dementia' to describe common symptoms – such as memory loss, confusion, and problems with speech and understanding – that get worse over time.

Dementia can affect a person at any age but it's more common in people over the age of 65.

There are many different types, subtypes and causes of dementia. The most common are Alzheimer's disease, vascular dementia, Lewy body dementia, frontotemporal dementia and mixed dementia.

There are currently around one million people in the UK with a diagnosis of dementia – and almost all of us will know someone living with the condition. Our dementia specialist Admiral Nurses explain the facts you need to know.

Alzheimer's disease?

Alzheimer's disease is the most common type of dementia in the UK. It's caused by a build-up of proteins in the brain which damage the brain cells' ability to transmit messages.

The symptoms of Alzheimer's disease tend to get worse over time. They include:

- difficulty remembering recent events (often retaining a good memory for past events)
- poor concentration
- difficulty recognising people or objects
- poor organisational skills
- confusion
- disorientation
- slow, muddled or repetitive speech
- difficulty performing everyday tasks such as cooking, paying bills, and shopping
- problems with decision-making

There is no cure for Alzheimer's disease, but medication is available to help slow its progression.

Vascular dementia

Vascular dementia is the second most common type of dementia. It's caused by problems in the supply of blood to the brain, commonly due to strokes or 'mini strokes' called transient ischaemic attacks (TIAs). This causes areas of cell damage in the brain.

Changes in a person's condition as a result of TIAs or a larger stroke are often sudden and then plateau (level off). But the damage caused often means the person never functions quite the same as they did before.

Vascular damage can also take place in the smaller vessels of the brain ('small vessel disease') and symptoms may be more gradual.

The symptoms of vascular dementia are often similar to Alzheimer's disease, such as memory problems, disorientation and difficulty with communication.

However, symptoms can depend on which area of the brain has been affected and may include specific problems with:

- language
- reading
- writing
- sudden changes in mood
- walking
- bladder control

Lewy body dementia

Lewy body dementia is a progressive condition that affects movement and motor control (the ability to control voluntary movements for specific tasks, like walking, getting dressed and using cutlery). Memory is often less affected than with other types of dementia.

A person with dementia with Lewy bodies might:

- be prone to falls
- have sudden bouts of confusion
- have tremors (shaking or trembling, similar to Parkinson's disease)
- have trouble swallowing
- experience disrupted sleep patterns due to intense dreams/nightmares
- have visual (sight) and auditory (hearing) hallucinations
- shuffle when they walk

Frontotemporal dementia

Frontotemporal dementia affects the frontal lobes of the brain: the part that controls behaviour, learning, personality and emotions.

It can affect people of all ages, but is more common in people aged 45 to 65 years than in those aged 65 and over.

Frontotemporal dementia can be difficult to diagnose. It's sometimes confused with depression, stress, anxiety, psychosis or obsessive compulsive disorder (OCD).

Frontotemporal dementia can cause inappropriate social behaviour and a lack of inhibitions. Eating patterns can also be affected, with people suddenly bingeing on food, especially sweet foods.

Mixed dementia

It's possible to have two types of dementia at the same time, most commonly Alzheimer's disease and vascular dementia.

person with mixed dementia will experience a mixture of ıe symptoms associated with the types of dementia they ave.

What is young onset dementia?

oung onset dementia is any type of dementia where ymptoms develop before the age of 65. You might hear it escribed as 'early onset dementia' or 'working age dementia.' 's thought that about 5% of people with dementia have oung onset dementia.

he most common types of dementia amongst younger eople are Alzheimer's disease, vascular dementia and ontotemporal dementia. Rare and genetically inherited ypes of dementia like Parkinson's and Huntington's disease re also more common in younger people.

roblems with language, vision, behaviour and/or ersonality may be the first symptoms, rather than memory oss. This can result in a delay in diagnosis as the symptoms ıay be wrongly attributed to another problem such as epression, work stress or relationship difficulties.

Getting a diagnosis of dementia

someone has symptoms of dementia, visit a GP as oon as possible. Some other treatable conditions have imilar symptoms, including infections, thyroid problems, irculatory issues, vitamin deficiency, sleep apnoea, stress nd depression, and it's important to rule these out.

he GP should take the person's medical and family history nd ask questions about their concentration, short-term nemory, mood, and behaviour changes.

he GP may then request blood tests, an MRI or CT scan to xamine the structure of the brain, and/or a chest X-ray to heck for any chest conditions that could be causing the ymptoms.

hey may also refer the person to a memory service/clinic, r to a specialist for further investigation, assessment and ossible treatment.

Your dementia questions answered

Why does dementia affect each person so differently?

he brain is made up of four lobes: frontal, temporal, arietal and occipital. Each lobe has a different function and epending on which part is damaged by dementia, it can ead to different signs and symptoms.

rontal lobes control:

- emotional expression
- personality
- problem-solving
- judgement
- motor function
- language
- motivation
- social behaviour

Temporal lobes control:

- memory
- speech
- language comprehension
- auditory (hearing) and visual perception
- emotional responses
- face recognition

Parietal lobes control:

- learnt skills such as reading, writing, calculations and driving
- object recognition
- spatial awareness

Occipital lobes control:

- spatial awareness
- colour recognition
- object recognition
- hand-eye coordination such as picking up items

How can I avoid getting dementia?

You can't prevent dementia, but there are things that could reduce your risk of developing it:

- eat a healthy, balanced diet
- if you're a smoker, stop smoking
- avoid drinking too much alcohol
- ask your GP to test your blood pressure and cholesterol level, and take advice on reducing these if they're raised
- stay physically and mentally active: activities like walking, gardening, singing, art, music, reading, puzzles and learning a new language may help

Is dementia hereditary?

Most dementias are not inherited, although Alzheimer's disease may be more likely if you have a family history of the condition. Genetics are also thought be involved in around 10% of young onset dementia cases. Some rarer causes of dementia can be inherited, like Huntington's disease.

Why is the number of people with dementia in the UK increasing?

There are over 900,000 people living with dementia in the UK and this is set to rise to over one million by 2025.

As awareness of dementia is increasing, people are more likely to recognise the signs and go to their GP to get a diagnosis.

People are also living for longer, and the risk of developing dementia gradually increases in people over the age of 65: one in six people in their 80s will develop dementia, and over one in three people aged 90 and over.

March 2023

Dementia: five charts that help explain Britain's biggest killer

From a diagnosis lottery to a spiralling bill we look at the UK's battle with the disease.

By Michael Goodier and Raphael Boyd

The number of people living with dementia in England is at an all-time high, with close to half a million diagnosed cases as of June 2024.

Dementia – Britain's biggest killer – is an umbrella term for many conditions and affects more than 55 million people worldwide. In England, about 7,000 people are diagnosed every month.

The global health cost is expected to almost triple by 2050, and is expected to reach $2.8 trillion by 2030.

Here we look at the nationwide fight against a pernicious disease.

It is Britain's biggest killer

Dementia is Britain's leading cause of death, with more people dying of the condition in England and Wales than from any other cause. In Scotland it is second only to coronary heart disease.

Although men are still slightly more likely to die from coronary heart disease than dementia across England and Wales, figures show dementia has been the biggest killer o women every year since 2012.

Dementia is the leading cause of death in England and Wales

Percentage of deaths, 2022

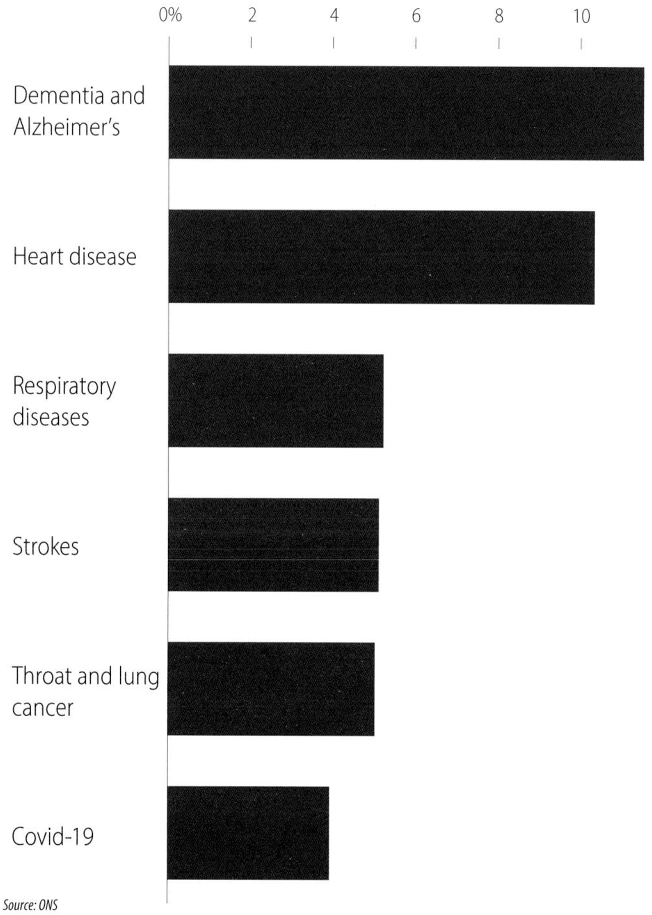

Source: ONS

A postcode lottery for diagnosis

Where you live can affect how likely you are to be diagnose with the condition. According to estimates, 65% of over-65 with dementia in England had been diagnosed as of Jun 2024 – while some areas of the country had rates as low a 46%.

The government has a target to diagnose 66.7% of patient However, the latest figures show 180 council areas in Englan are below that figure. The target was last met nationwide i 2019.

Last year, a report from the all-party parliamentary grou on dementia found that structural issues could be stoppin patients seeking or obtaining a diagnosis. These include access to a GP, cultural barriers, waiting times for memor assessment, lack of post-diagnostic support and insufficien scanners.

London – the youngest region in England – has by far th fewest number of cases compared with its population, wit only 0.6% of residents confirmed to be living with dementi The highest number of cases was found in the regions wit the oldest populations – the north-east, south-east an south-west.

In 2021, Alzheimer's Society UK predicted that there wer almost 900,000 people living with dementia, with about ha of those cases thought to be misdiagnosed or not picke up at all. A total 66,000 of those thought to have dementi lived in Scotland, with 44,000 living in Wales and 22,000 i Northern Ireland.

It is not a disease that just affects older people

Although almost everyone diagnosed is over the age of 65 one in every 14 known dementia sufferers in England i mid-2024 had young-onset dementia, meaning they wer diagnosed before their 65th birthday.

Men are more likely to be diagnosed with young-onse dementia than women. NHS figures show there were 13% more men than women under the age of 65 diagnosed wit dementia, and almost double the number of men under 50 than women under 50 with a diagnosis in England.

Looking at older age groups, women with dementi outnumber men and from the age of 80 there are twice a many women with the disease as there are men – probabl because women have a longer life expectancy. NHS figure also suggest that white people have a lower rate of diagnosi than other ethnic groups.

Dementia diagnosis rates are geographically unequal

Percentage of people estimated to have dementia who have a recorded diagnosis

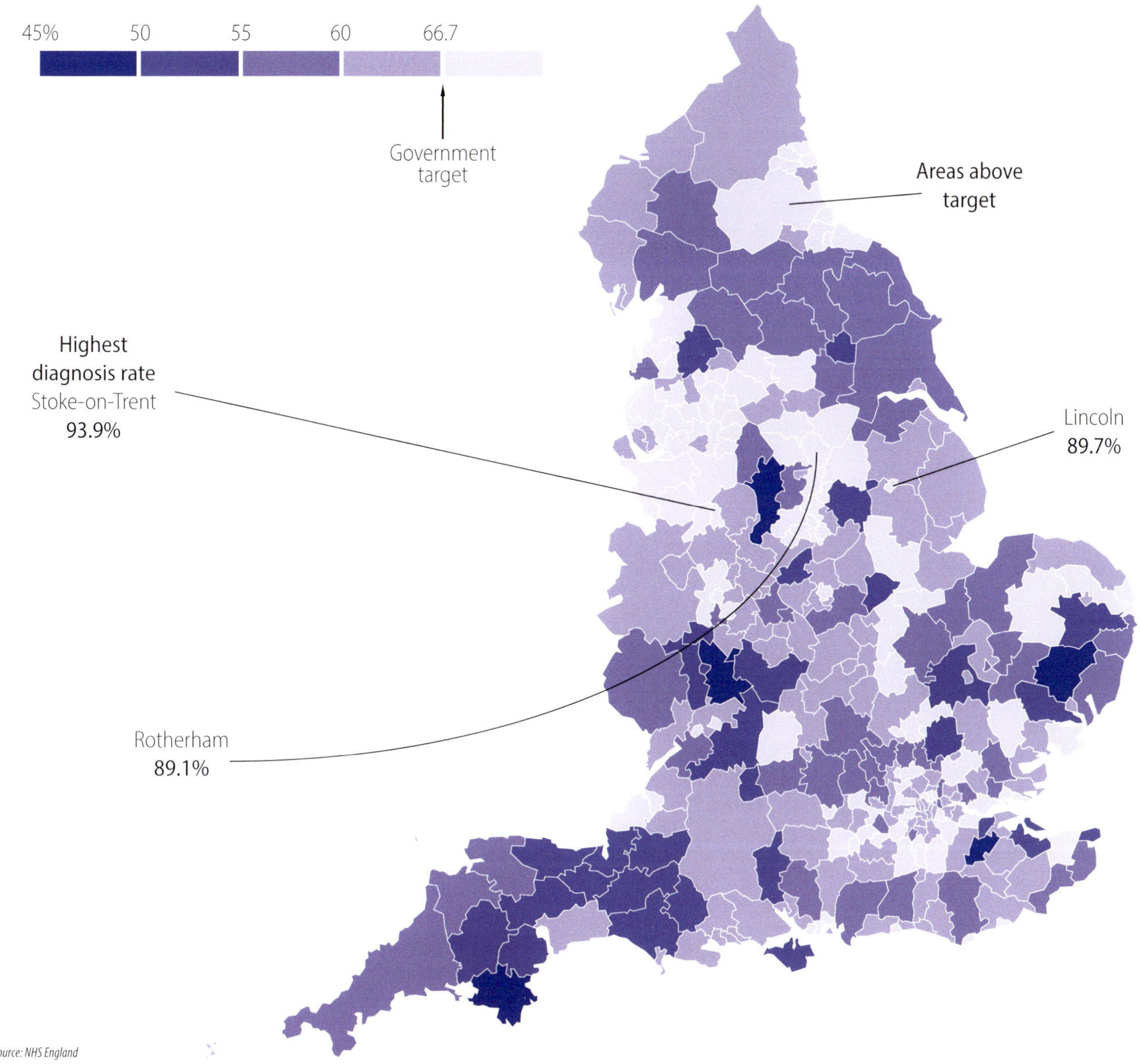

Source: NHS England

A record 487,432 people in England have a dementia diagnosis

Recorded dementia diagnosis in England, June 2024, thousands

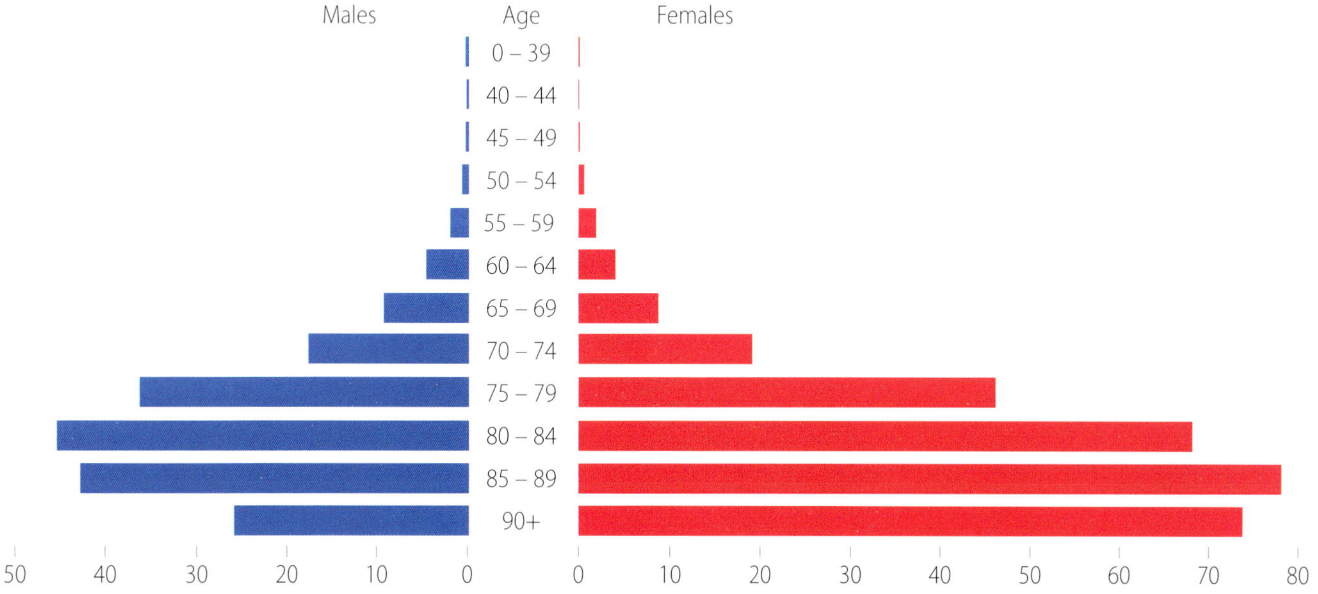

ource: NHS England

Ageing populations will lead to dementia cases rising globally

Estimated number of people with dementia per 1,000 population, selected G20 countries

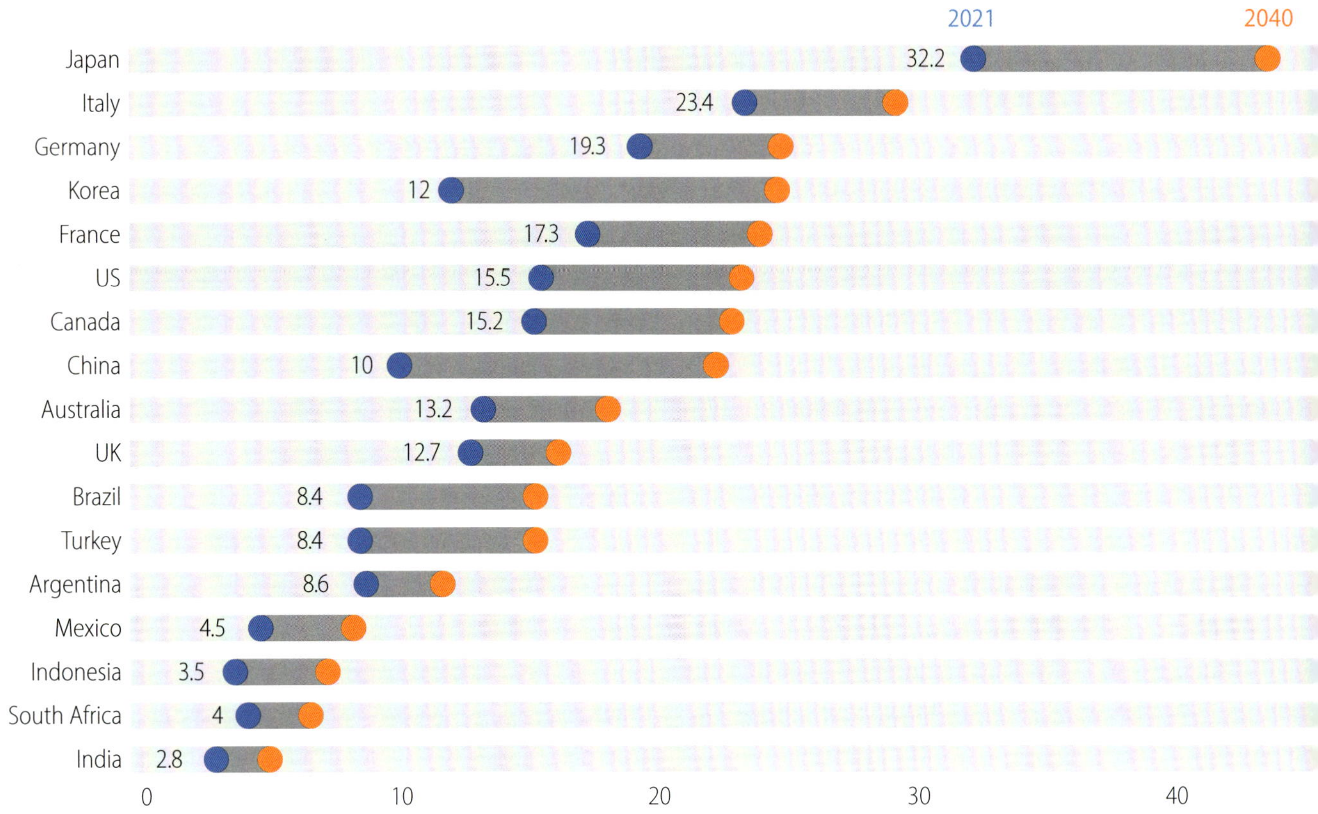

Source: Source: OECD analysis of data from the World Alzheimer Report 2015 and the United Nations World Population Prospects

Alzheimer's is the most commonly diagnosed form of dementia

Number of recorded diagnoses by type, England

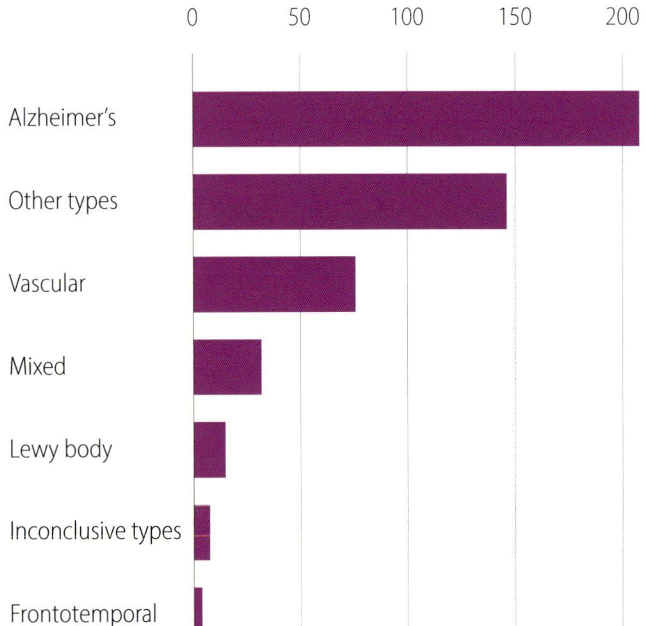

Source: NHS England

There are many kinds of dementia

Alzheimer's is by far the most commonly diagnosed type of dementia, making up 42.4% of diagnoses in England and about 62% in Scotland. In England, the next most common types of dementia are vascular dementia (15.6%) and mixed dementia, where a patient has more than one type.

However, the diagnosis figures don't represent the fu picture. Hundreds of thousands of people with certai types of dementia, especially Lewy bodies, which include Parkinson's disease dementia, may be living without diagnosis.

A global issue with a rising healthcare bill

The number of dementia cases globally is expected to tripl by 2050, as the world's population grows and ages.

A 2022 study in the Lancet predicted that the number c people with dementia would increase from 57 million case worldwide in 2019 to 153 million by 2050 – with increase in sub-Saharan Africa driven by population growth, an increases in east Asian mainly driven by population ageing

With a rising caseload comes a rising healthcare bill. Thi year a study for the Alzheimer's Society found that the cos of the disease in the UK alone, including economic impact is likely to more than double from £42.5 billion today t £90.6 billion by 2040.

Globally, costs are expected to double even sooner – fror $1.3 trillion a year in 2019 to $2.8 trillion by 2030. It may b Britain's biggest killer, but dementia is also an urgent globa issue that policymakers and public health planners aroun the world will have to engage with.

14 August 2024

Brain function of older adults catching up with younger generations

The brain function of older generations is improving, with the gap between old and young healthy adults lessening, according to research by Nottingham Trent University.

By Helen Breese

The three-part study reviewed evidence from 60 independent research papers regarding cognition in older and younger adults to explore trends and determine whether age differences are changing over time.

It also examined the results of a study by lead researcher Dr Stephen Badham, Associate Professor in Psychology at NTU's School of Social Sciences, which assessed and compared the cognitive abilities of more than 1,000 older and younger adults at different points in time.

Cognition relates to how the brain processes information and can be linked to education, physical activity, and diet quality. It is also a factor in diagnosing age-related diseases such as dementia.

The studies in the review examined the cognition of older adults over time, particularly comparing earlier-born adults with later-born adults. The research also explored whether an age-related reduction in brain function is changing over time by analysing historic studies that compared young and older adults.

Some of the factors measured included verbal fluency, for example the ability to list words within a category; memory, such as delayed recall, delayed recognition, immediate memory and working memory; and cognitive speed.

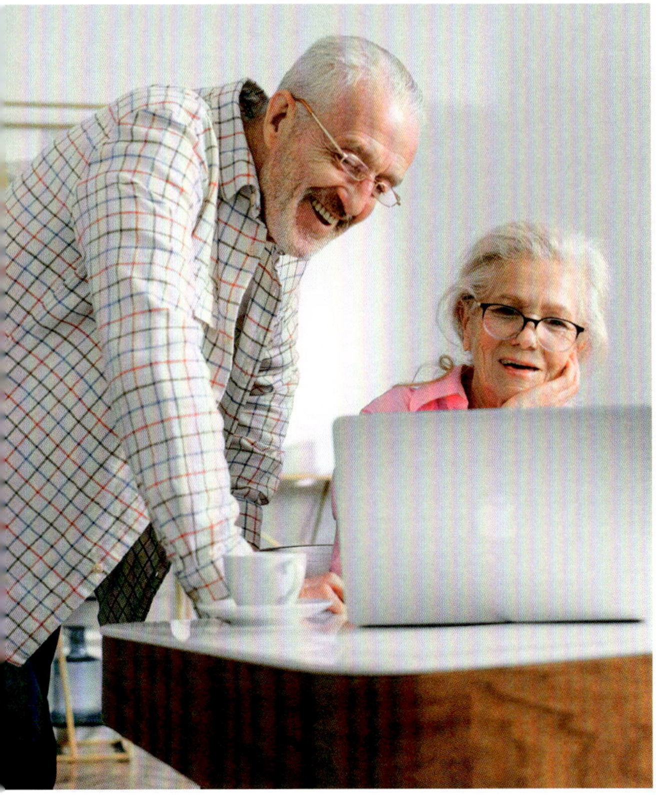

The evidence points overall to improving and higher cognitive performance among older adults with 83 of the measures used (68%) across the studies showing better performance in later cohorts of older adults than earlier cohorts, only six (5%) showed the reverse.

In contrast, findings show that young adults' cognition remained relatively flat across time – closing the gap between generations.

The findings were linked to ongoing improvements in education, healthcare, nutrition and access to more mentally stimulating, digital environments, which might have previously applied mainly to younger adults.

Associate Professor Stephen Badham said: 'Much existing research shows that IQ has been improving globally throughout the 20th century. This means that later-born generations are more cognitively able than those born earlier.

'However, there is growing evidence that time-based increases in IQ are levelling off, such that in the most recent couple of decades, young adults are no more cognitively able than those born shortly beforehand. As a result, the current data show that young adult advantages in cognition relative to older adults, such as memory ability and speed of processing, are now getting smaller over time. This means that when we compare young and older adults today, the gap is smaller than it was in the past.

'Therefore, the decline an individual might expect to experience as they become older is smaller than originally thought. In other words, we can expect to be more cognitively able than our grandparents were when we reach their age.

'Finally, as older adults are performing better in general than previous generations, it may be necessary to revise definitions of dementia that depend on an individual's expected level of ability. This is because dementia is defined as cognitive ability that is below normal and the current results suggest that as healthy older adults become more cognitively able, we may need to revise our definition of normal when diagnosing dementia.'

24 April 2024

The full paper *The older population is more cognitively able than in the past and age-related deficits in cognition are diminishing over time* can be read in the journal *Developmental Review*.

www.ntu.ac.uk

Here's a simple, science-backed way to sharpen your thinking and improve your memory

An article from The Conversation.

By Ben Singh, Research Fellow, Allied Health & Human Performance, University of South Australia and Ashleigh E. Smith, Associate Professor, Healthy Ageing, University of South Australia

Many of us turn to Sudoku, Wordle or brain-training apps to sharpen our minds. But research is increasingly showing one of the best ways to boost memory, focus and brain health is exercise.

Our new research reviewed data from more than 250,000 participants across 2,700 studies. We found exercise helps boost brain function – whether it's walking, cycling, yoga, dancing, or even playing active video games such as Pokémon GO.

Moving your body improves how we think, make decisions, remember things and stay focused – no matter your age.

What the science says

Our review adds to a growing body of research that shows regular physical activity improves three key areas of brain function:

- cognition, which is your overall ability to think clearly, learn and make decisions
- memory, especially short-term memory and the ability to remember personal experiences
- executive function, which includes focus, planning, problem-solving and managing emotions.

We conducted an umbrella review, which means we looked at the results of more than 130 high-quality research reviews that had already combined findings from many exercise studies. These studies usually involved people starting a new, structured exercise program, not just tracking the exercise they were already doing.

To assess the effects on cognition, memory and executive function, the original studies used a range of brain function tests. These included things like remembering word lists, solving puzzles, or quickly switching between tasks – simple activities designed to reliably measure how well the brain is working.

The improvements were small to moderate. On average, exercise led to a noticeable boost in cognition, with slightly smaller but still meaningful gains in memory and executive function.

The benefits showed up across all age groups, thoug children and teens saw major gains in memory.

People with attention-deficit hyperactivity disorder (ADHD showed greater improvements in executive function afte physical activity than other population groups.

The brain started responding fairly quickly – many peopl experienced improvements after just 12 weeks of startin regular exercise.

Generally, the greatest benefits were seen in those doin at least 30 minutes of exercise on most days of the week aiming for a total of about 150 minutes per week.

What's happening in the brain?

Activities such as walking or cycling can increase the siz of the hippocampus, the part of the brain responsible fo memory and learning.

In one study, older adults who did aerobic exercise for a yea grew their hippocampus by 2%, effectively reversing one t two years of age-related brain shrinkage.

More intense workouts, such as running or high-intensit interval training, can further boost neuroplasticity – th brain's ability to adapt and rewire itself. This helps you lear more quickly, think more clearly and stay mentally shar with age.

Another reason to get moving

The world's population is ageing. By 2030, one in six o people will be aged over 60. With that comes a rising risk o dementia, Alzheimer's disease and cognitive decline.

At the same time, many adults aren't moving enough. On in three adults aren't meeting the recommended levels o physical activity.

Adults should aim for at least 150 minutes of moderat exercise – such as brisk walking – each week, or at least 7 minutes of more vigorous activity, like running.

It's also important to incorporate muscle-strengthenin exercises, such as lifting weights, into workouts at leas twice a week.

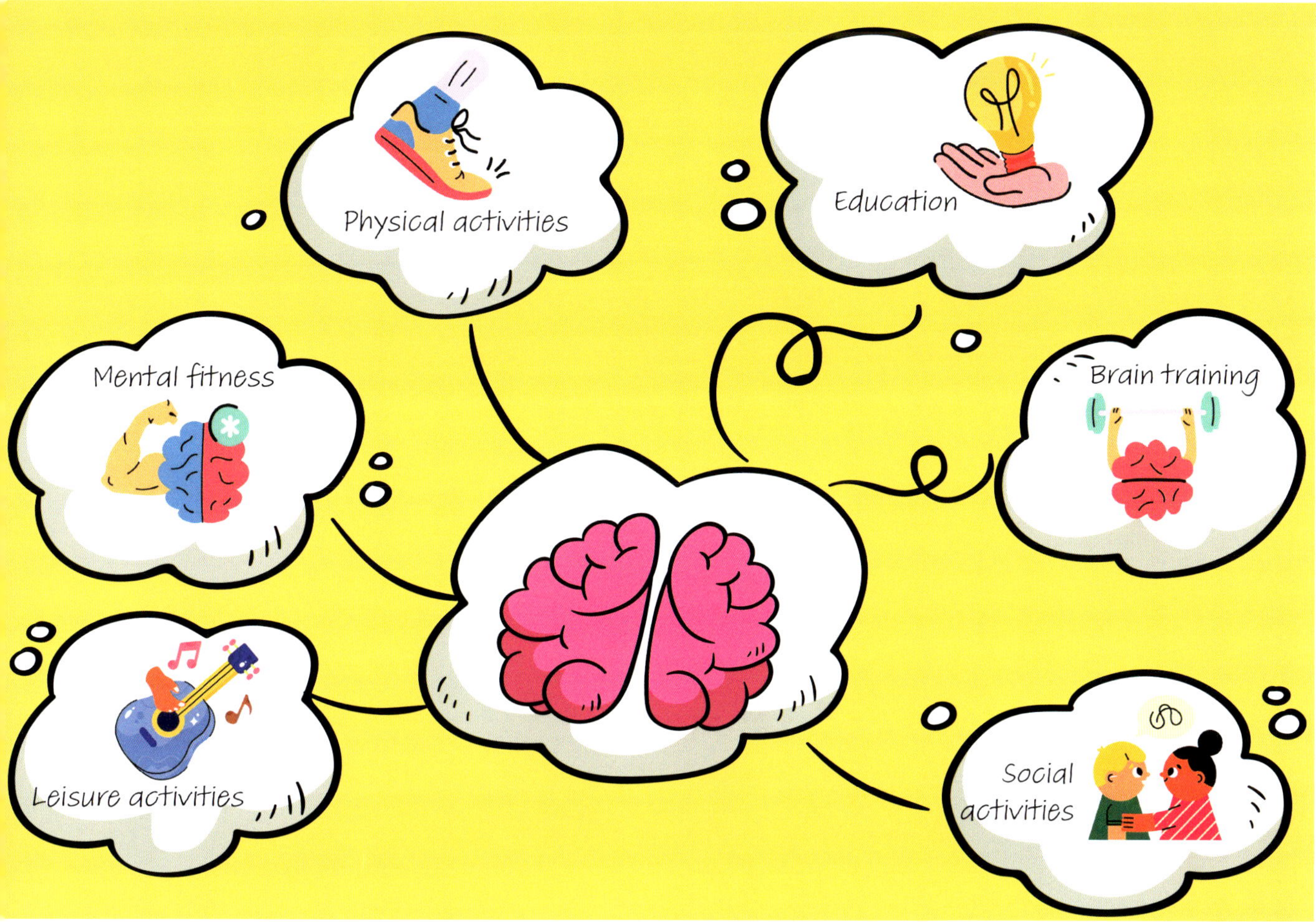

Everyday movement counts

ou don't need to run marathons or lift heavy weights to enefit. Our study showed lower-intensity activities such s yoga, tai chi and 'exergames' (active video games) can be ust as effective – sometimes even more so.

hese activities engage both the brain and body. Tai chi, or instance, requires focus, coordination and memorising equences.

xergames often include real-time decision-making and apid response to cues. This trains attention and memory.

mportantly, these forms of movement are inclusive. They an be done at home, outdoors, or with friends, making hem a great option for people of all fitness levels or those vith limited mobility.

lthough you may already be doing a lot through daily life · like walking instead of driving or carrying shopping bags ome – it's still important to find time for structured exercise, uch as lifting weights at the gym or doing a regular yoga lass, to get the full benefits for your brain and body.

Real-life applications

f you're a grandparent, consider playing Wii Sports virtual ennis or bowling with your grandchild. If you're a teenager vith signs of ADHD, try a dance class, and see if it impacts our concentration in class. If you're a busy parent, you night be more clear-headed if you can squeeze a 20-minute oga video session between meetings.

In each of these cases, you're not just being active, you're giving your brain a valuable tune-up. And unlike most brain-training apps or supplements, exercise delivers far reaching benefits, including improved sleep and mental health.

Workplaces and schools are starting to take note. Short movement breaks are being introduced during the workday to improve employee focus.

Schools that incorporate physical activity into the classroom are seeing improvements in students' attention and academic performance.

Exercise is one of the most powerful and accessible tools we have for supporting brain health. Best of all, it's free, widely available and it's never too late to start.

8 April 2025

Chapter 3

Wellness in Old Age

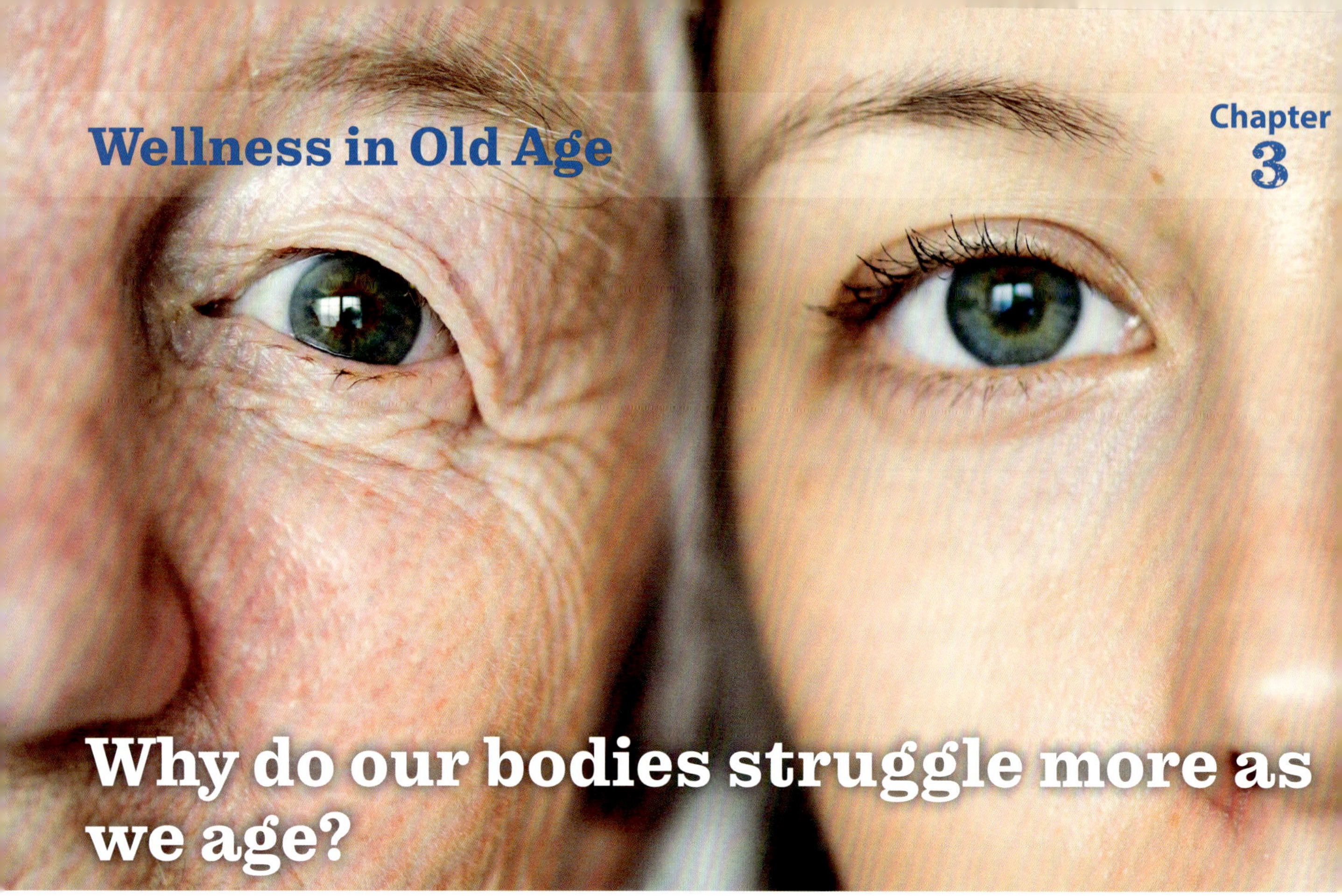

Why do our bodies struggle more as we age?

Ageing is a natural part of life – a journey every human experiences in one way or another. As we grow older, our bodies and minds go through gradual changes that can affect how we feel, move, and function. While many of these changes are completely normal, they also mean that older adults are more likely to face a range of health issues.

So, what exactly makes elderly people more prone to illness and injury? The answer lies in a combination of biology, lifetime habits, environmental factors, and the natural wear and tear on the body. This article explores why ageing increases vulnerability to health problems – and what we can do about it.

Natural ageing

As we age, our bodies gradually slow down. This is a biological process called natural or intrinsic ageing. It involves a decline in cell function, slower regeneration of tissues, and changes to organs and systems throughout the body.

You might notice wrinkles forming, skin becoming thinner, or joints feeling stiffer. Bones become less dense, and muscles naturally shrink if they are not used. Our metabolism slows down, and hormone levels such as oestrogen and testosterone decrease. The heart and lungs may not work quite as efficiently, and the brain can take slightly longer to process information.

None of these changes mean that someone is 'unwell' – they are simply part of growing older. However, they can make it easier for illnesses or injuries to take hold.

Lifetime exposures

Our environment and lifestyle choices throughout life ca have a huge impact on how we age. This includes bot harmful exposures and helpful habits. The longer we ar exposed to certain risks, the more they can contribute t age-related health issues.

Pollution is one example. Air pollution, especially in urba areas, can damage the lungs and heart over time. Breathin in harmful particles every day, even at low levels, adds u across the years.

Unhealthy habits also take a toll. Smoking, drinking alcoho eating poorly, or not exercising can lead to long-tern damage. These behaviours can increase the risk of hear disease, stroke, diabetes, and more.

Sun exposure is another factor. Ultraviolet (UV) rays from th sun can cause premature ageing of the skin and increase th risk of skin cancer. Without sun protection, years of exposur can leave lasting damage.

Even chronic stress can contribute to ageing. Constan pressure or emotional strain affects the immune system blood pressure, and mental health.

Chronic conditions and weaker immunity

As people age, the immune system becomes less effective This is known as immunosenescence – a natural weakenin of the body's defence system. It means older adults are mor vulnerable to infections and take longer to recover fron illness or injury.

Inflammation in the body also tends to increase with age. While inflammation is a normal part of healing, chronic inflammation can lead to serious conditions such as heart disease, arthritis, and Alzheimer's disease.

In addition, older adults are more likely to live with chronic conditions – long-term illnesses such as high blood pressure, diabetes, or osteoporosis. These conditions are not always caused by age, but ageing makes them more likely and harder to manage.

Common health issues in older adults

While everyone experiences ageing differently, certain health problems become more common later in life. Understanding them can help people seek the right support, make informed decisions, and take action to protect their wellbeing – both now and in the future. The choices we make today, from how we eat and move to how we manage stress, can play a big role in shaping our health as we grow older.

Arthritis

Arthritis is one of the most widespread conditions in older adults. Osteoarthritis, the most common type, causes the cartilage in joints to wear away. This leads to pain, stiffness, and reduced mobility – often in the knees, hips, hands, or spine. Although arthritis can't be cured, treatments such as physiotherapy, medication, and surgery can improve quality of life.

Diabetes

Type 2 diabetes becomes more common with age, especially in people who are overweight or physically inactive. It develops when the body can no longer regulate blood sugar levels effectively. If left untreated, it can lead to serious complications such as stroke, nerve damage, heart disease, and kidney problems. The good news is that healthy lifestyle choices – like eating a balanced diet, staying active, and maintaining a healthy weight – can help prevent or delay the onset of type 2 diabetes. In some cases, these changes may even reverse the condition. However, some people may also need medication to manage their blood sugar levels effectively.

Eyesight and hearing

Vision and hearing often change with age. Conditions like cataracts, macular degeneration, and glaucoma affect many older adults, making reading or driving more difficult. Age-related hearing loss (presbycusis) is also very common and can impact communication and social engagement. Regular check-ups and the use of glasses or hearing aids can make a big difference.

Cancer

The risk of developing cancer increases with age, largely because of the gradual build-up of changes to cells over time. Some of the most common cancers in older people include skin cancer, breast cancer, prostate cancer, and bowel cancer. Early detection through regular screening can improve outcomes.

Cognitive health

It's natural for memory to become a little slower with age, but significant confusion or forgetfulness can be a sign of dementia. Alzheimer's disease is the most common type. While there is no cure, early support, brain training, and social interaction can help people live well for longer.

Mental health

Older people may face mental health challenges due to bereavement, isolation, or physical decline. Depression and anxiety are often overlooked in older adults, especially when symptoms are mistaken for normal ageing. It's important to remember that emotional wellbeing is just as important as physical health.

Bladder and bowel issues

Problems such as incontinence (loss of bladder control) and constipation are more common with age. These can result from weaker pelvic muscles, side effects of medication, or underlying health conditions. Though embarrassing for some to discuss, they are very common and treatable with medical support.

Respiratory illnesses

Older lungs are less efficient, making conditions like chronic obstructive pulmonary disease (COPD) more likely, especially among former smokers. Recovery from colds, flu, and pneumonia can also take longer. Vaccines and breathing exercises can help prevent complications.

Physical injury and frailty

As muscles shrink and bones lose strength, older people become more prone to falls and fractures. Frailty is a condition where the body loses strength and resilience, making it harder to recover from illness or injury. Weight-bearing exercises, good nutrition, and home safety adaptations can reduce these risks.

So why are older people more prone to health issues? It's a combination of biology, environment, and experience. The body changes naturally with age, but those changes are influenced by everything we've been exposed to and how we've looked after ourselves along the way.

That said, ageing is not all decline. Many older adults live full and active lives, especially when they prioritise healthy habits, stay socially connected, and get regular medical care. Understanding the changes that come with age helps us face them with confidence – and support ourselves and others to live well, no matter our age.

Scientists study world's oldest person to unearth secret to long life

Maria Branyas, the oldest woman in the world at 116, has agreed to help Spanish scientists.

By Amelia Neath

Scientists are studying the world's oldest person to try to unearth the secret to a long life, after being bewildered by the 'super grandmother's' great health at 116 years old.

Maria Branyas was born in San Fransisco in 1907 but returned to Spain when she was eight and settled in Catalonia.

Ms Branyas, known to her X followers as the 'Super Catalan Grandma', has lived in the region ever since and has resided in the same nursing home, Residència Santa María del Tura, for the last 22 years, according to the *Guinness World Records*.

Now, the world record holder has agreed to undergo scientific testing – which researchers hope will further their understanding of certain illnesses associated with old age, such as neurodegenerative or cardiovascular diseases.

Despite her age, Ms Branyas has no health complications other than hearing and mobility issues and still has a great memory.

'She has a completely lucid head,' scientist Manel Esteller told ABC, a Spanish outlet. 'She remembers with impressive clarity episodes of her when she was only four years old, and she does not present any cardiovascular disease, common in elderly people.'

Mr Esteller, a well-renowned Spanish scientist focusing on genetics and how they apply to health conditions, recently came across Ms Branyas and was curious how her genetic makeup might affect her ageing.

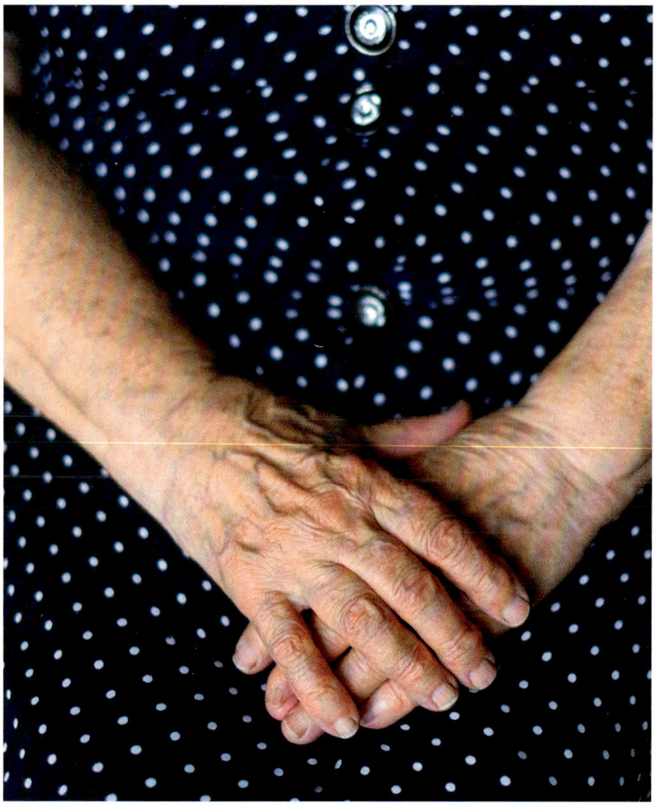

After a long talk with Ms Branyas, Mr Esteller believes there must be more to her longevity than meets the eye.

The remarkable woman has not had an easy life; she survived an earthquake while she was in the US, a major fire, both world wars, the Spanish Civil War, the Spanish Flu pandemic and, more recently, survived COVID-19 in 2020.

Ms Branyas lost her father when she was very young while the family were on a ship from the US to Spain; he died of pulmonary tuberculosis, the *Guinness World Record* reports.

On top of losing her father, she suffered permanent hearing loss in one ear while on board the ship after falling while playing with her brothers.

Despite the various pandemics, wars and family loss she has endured, her longevity has made scientists questioning what her secret could be.

'We know Maria's chronological age, 116 years, but we must determine her biological age,' Mr Esteller said to ABC believing that 'she is much younger' physically.

The scientist has taken biological samples of saliva, blood and urine from Ms Branyas, which are thought to be the 'longest-lived' biological samples and have great scientific value, Josep Carreras, the head of a leukaemia research institute, said to ABC.

The samples will be compared with the 116-year-old's middle daughter, who is 79 years old.

Ms Branyas often has been asked what her secret is to her long life, and she uses her X account to post her advice for others.

She attributed her longevity to 'order, tranquillity, good connection with family and friends, contact with nature, emotional stability, no worries, no regrets, lots of positivity and staying away from toxic people'.

However, she also credits a great amount of luck.

'It is clear that there is a genetic component because there are several members of her family who are over 90 years old,' Mr Esteller said.

The rare biological samples will assess her genes, which will hopefully advance the research of drugs that could help diseases associated with age and cancer.

As for Ms Branyas, she said on her X account that she is 'very happy [she] can be useful for research and progress'.

26 October 2023

Older adults who remain more active have a better quality of life, study finds

A reduction in the amount of time spent physically active when adults are over 60 years old is linked to lower quality of life, a Cambridge study of almost 1,500 adults has shown.

The same was also true for increases in the amount of sedentary time, such as watching TV or reading. The researchers say this highlights the need to encourage older adults to remain active.

Physical activity – particularly when it is moderate-intensity and raises your heart rate – is known to reduce the risk of a number of diseases, including heart disease, stroke, diabetes and cancer. The NHS recommends that adults do at least 150 minutes of moderate-intensity activity or 75 minutes of vigorous-intensity activity a week. Older adults are also recommended to break up prolonged periods of being sedentary with light activity when physically possible, or at least with standing, as this has distinct health benefits for older people.

A team led by researchers at the University of Cambridge examined activity levels among 1,433 participants aged 60 and above using accelerometers. The participants had been recruited to the EPIC (European Prospective Investigation into Cancer)-Norfolk study.

Alongside this, the team also looked at health-related quality of life, a measure of health and wellbeing that includes pain, ability to care for yourself and anxiety/mood. Participants were given a score between 0 (worst quality of life) and 1 (best) based on their responses to a questionnaire. Lower quality of life scores are linked with an increased risk of hospitalisation, worse outcomes following hospitalisation, and early death.

Participants were followed up an average of just under six years later to look at changes in their behaviour and quality of life. The results of the study are published in *Health and Quality of Life Outcomes.*

On average, six years after their first assessment, both men and women were doing around 24 minutes less moderate-to-vigorous physical activity per day. At the same time, the total sedentary time increased by an average of around 33 minutes a day for men and around 38 minutes a day for women.

Those individuals who did more moderate-to-vigorous physical activity and spent less time sedentary at their first assessment had a higher quality of life later on. An hour a day spent more active was associated with a 0.02 higher quality of life score.

For every minute a day less of moderate-to-vigorous physical activity measured six years after the first assessment, quality of life scores dropped by 0.03. This means that an individual who spent 15 minutes a day less engaged in such activity would have seen their score drop by 0.45.

Increases in sedentary behaviours were also associated with poorer quality of life – a drop in the score of 0.012 for everyone minute a day increase in total sedentary time six years after the first measurement. This means that an individual who spent 15 minutes a day more sitting down would have seen their score drop by 0.18.

To put the results into a clinical context, a 0.1 point improvement in quality of life scores has previously been associated with a 6.9% reduction in early death and a 4.2% reduction in risk of hospitalisation.

Dr Dharani Yerrakalva from the Department of Public Health and Primary Care at the University of Cambridge said: 'Keeping yourself active and limiting – and where you can, breaking up – the amount of time you spend sitting down is really important whatever stage of life you're at. This seems to be particularly important in later life, when it can lead to potentially significant improvements to your quality of life and your physical and mental wellbeing.'

Because the team measured physical activity and sedentary behaviour at different points of time, they say they can be reasonably confident that they have shown a causal link – that is, that quality of life improves because people remain more physically active, for example.

Dr Yerrakalva added: 'There are several ways in which improvements in our physical behaviours might help maintain a better quality of life. For example, more physical activity reduces pain in common conditions such as osteoarthritis, and we know that being more physically active improves muscle strength which allows older adults to continue to care for themselves. Similarly, depression and anxiety are linked to quality of life, and can be improved by being more active and less sedentary.'

The EPIC-Norfolk study is funded by the Medical Research Council and Cancer Research UK.

Five ways to keep yourself physically active in older age

- A brisk daily walk – ideally for around 20 minutes
- Gardening
- A bicycle ride
- Dancing
- Tennis.

4 July 2023

www.cam.ac.uk

Four lifestyle habits that might just help you live to 100

An article from The Conversation.

By Bradley Elliot, Reader in Ageing Physiology, University of Westminster

A 115-year-old Surrey woman named Ethel Caterham has officially been handed the title of the oldest living human alive.

Many people reading this news may wonder what Caterham's secret is.

While it isn't usually a good idea to take health and longevity advice from supercentenarians (as they're often the exception rather than the rule), there are some lifestyle pointers that we can take from research on groups of long-lived people that might help us increase our chances of living a longer life.

1. Physical activity

Physical activity is good for you – who knew? Research shows that people who are more physically active each day tend to live longer, healthier lives. One study found that going from no physical activity to about 75 minutes per week of brisk walking increased life expectancy by about two years.

But perhaps less well known is just how bad inactivity is for your health and longevity. It's a tad difficult to explain, but the positive effects of exercise are actually different from the negative effects of inactivity. That means that you can have a positive influence on your health by being both more active and avoiding being inactive.

Yet as good as structured exercise is for you, it can't by itself offset the harms of inactivity and sitting all day. Research even shows that being sedentary is associated with higher risk of premature death from any cause.

If you want to live longer, you should try to avoid sitting for long periods of time if possible. Practical tips for this include

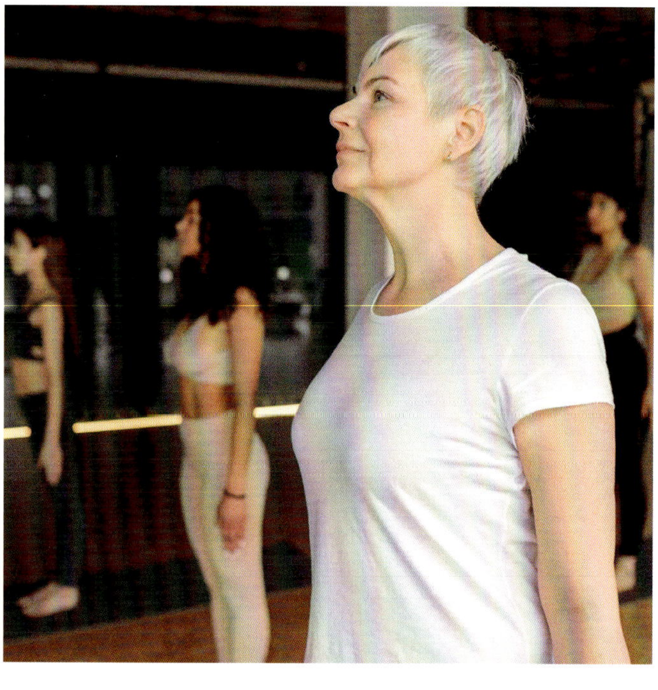

standing up every 30 minutes, going to see someone in the office instead of calling or emailing them and standing on public transport during commuting. This, plus the aim to do about 30 minutes moderate exercise most days will help maximise your odds of a long, healthy life.

2. Eat your veggies

The advice many kids dread: eat your vegetables if you want to live a long time.

A recent study that followed around 100,000 people over a 30 year period found that people who made it to 70 years of age in good health (meaning they had no chronic diseases) typically ate more fruits, vegetables, whole grains, nuts and

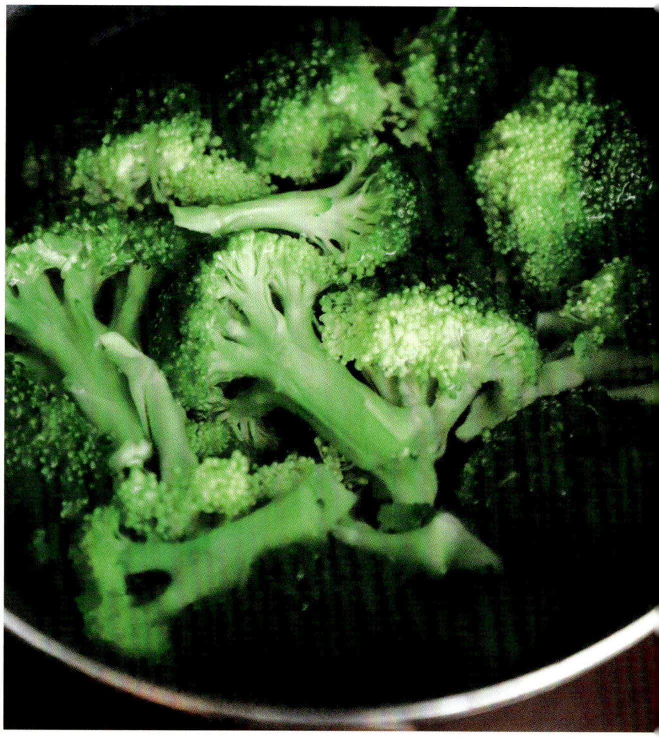

legumes, and fewer trans-fats, red or processed meats, fried foods and sugary foods. Importantly, this study doesn't say that you must be a vegan, or never eat red meats – it only identifies trends within diets associated with healthy ageing.

When and how much you eat may also play a role when it comes to ageing. Research on caloric restriction and intermittent fasting in animals has shown both can increase lifespan. Our preliminary work in humans has also shown that following a fasting diet for three weeks can cause similar, positive metabolic shifts that match what we've seen in animals that will live longer. However, larger studies over longer time frames are needed to establish effects on healthspan and lifespan in humans.

3. Sleep

Regular, good quality sleep is also important for lifelong health and overall longevity.

In a study of about 500,000 British people, irregular sleep patterns were associated with a 50% higher risk of early death compared to those with regular sleep patterns. Shift workers showed higher risk for strokes, and nurses who worked rotating shifts for decades were less healthy and had earlier deaths at retirement compared to nurses who didn't work shifts.

While this data suggests that good quality, regular sleep is important for good health, how much sleep you need and when you should go to bed appears to be highly individualistic. This makes giving population-wide recommendations difficult – which is why the NHS recommends adults get between 7–9 hours sleep.

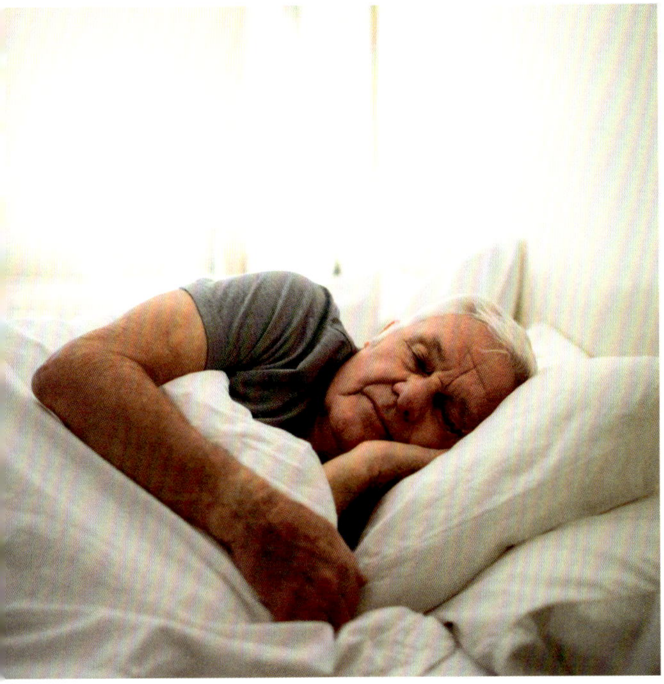

4. Stress

Stress has many effects on your health.

For instance, increasing evidence shows that early-life stressors (such as loss of a parent, neglect or abuse) can negatively affect health later in life – even down to a molecular and cellular level by increasing inflammation levels in ways that could increase the risk of poor health and premature death in older age.

Conversely, older adults that show increased psychological resilience to stress are less likely to die from any cause. As little as eight weeks of regular yoga is enough to improve psychological resilience in older adults.

Possibly linked is the effect of social connections. Those that live more socially active lives also tend to live longer. In fact, people over 65 who are socially active daily are three times more likely to live for five more years compared to those that almost never engage in social activities.

It's a common finding that strong social networks appear to enhance longevity. This may be due to the way social connections help us alleviate stressors in our lives.

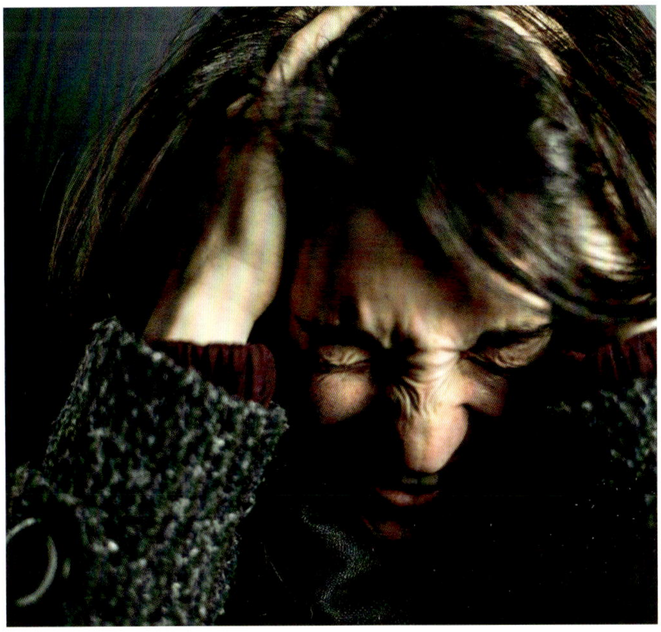

The role of genetics

While there are many lifestyle habits we can change, one thing we can't control when it comes to our lifespans is genetics. Some research suggests that naturally-occurring mutations in genes associated with longevity are more common in long-lived people.

Although it's hard to tease out the role of genetics versus lifestyle when it comes to lifespan, current predictions suggest that longevity is between 20–40% related to genetics.

But good genetics aren't everything. Although Ethel Caterham has made it to the remarkable age of 115 – and one of her sisters lived to be 104 – Caterham's two daughters pre-deceased her at 71 and 83 years of age.

And even if you do win the genetic jackpot and follow a good lifestyle, you would still be very lucky to make it to Caterham's grand old age of 115. Cells mutate, clots form, biological luck runs out. Still, if you want to maximise your odds of living longer and staying as healthy as possible, aim to be more physically active each day, eat a good diet, get a good night's sleep and keep stress levels low.

16 May 2025

How to live to 100 – which habit is most important?

In small groups, read and discuss the four healthy habits from the article.

Rank them from most to least important, and explain your reasons. Then, join another group and compare your rankings. Do you agree? Why or why not?

Two million older people now have some unmet need for social care

New Age UK report finds older people are often struggling due to insufficient access to high-quality NHS treatment, as well as social care, and that the system is currently under-preparec for population ageing.

Age UK strongly supports Lord Darzi's conclusion that the answer lies in focusing more or prevention and early intervention, supporting older people at home or in a care home to stay fit and well.

New analysis carried out by Age UK has found that 2 million older people in England are now living with some unmet need for social care.

This stark finding is one of many in a major new Age UK report, published today: *The State of Health and Care of Older People in 2024*. Drawing on the latest available data, the report concludes that England's health and care services continue to be under enormous pressure so that, despite the best efforts of many dedicated staff, they are currently unable to meet the needs of all the older people presenting who require treatment, care and support.

Long-standing problems were greatly exacerbated during the pandemic years and despite some recovery since then in some areas, in others it has not yet proved possible to arrest a decline in capacity, service availability and performance, with extremely worrying implications for older people and their families and unpaid carers. This is all the more concerning in light of a rising older population, the growth of which will accelerate still further over the next decade, increasing by a projected 4.3 million by 2044.

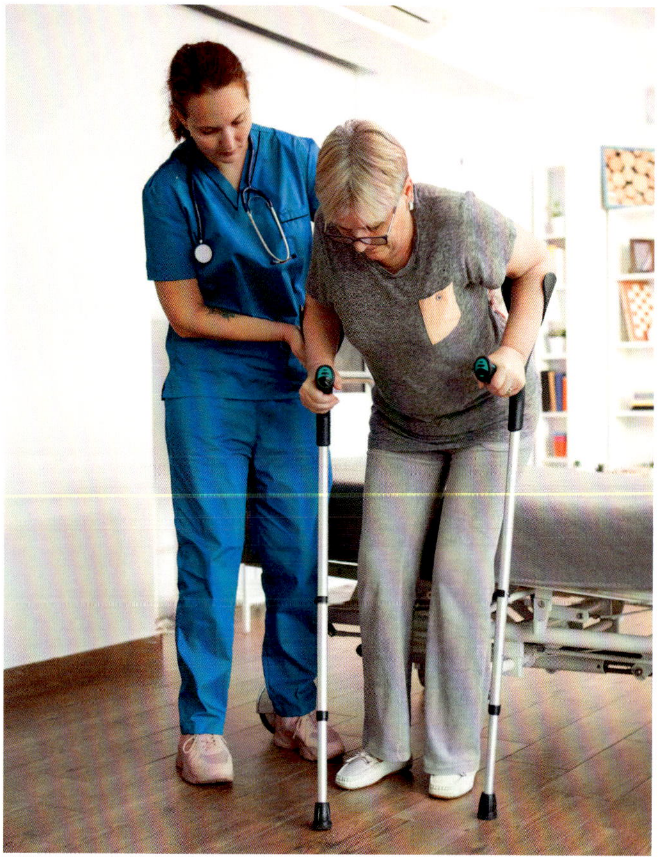

However, more optimistically, the new report shows that significant numbers of emergency hospital admissions could definitely be avoided if the right kind of help was provided earlier on, before relatively minor health problems develop into full scale crises. The inability of services to intervene quickly or effectively enough to support older people at home leads to many waiting for very long periods in A&E and then becoming stuck in a hospital bed because of a lack of community-based care, creating huge problems for hospital managers and undermining their own chances of making a good recovery.

Age UK finds that in particular, very old people aged over 80 are often not getting the good and timely NHS treatment, care and support they need and ought to be able to expect. More than one in four (28%) are living with some unmet need for social care, and people in this age group are also the most likely to experience long waits in A&E, having arrived there by ambulance. Many have complex health and care needs and at the moment the system is often insufficiently geared up to meeting them, though there are some isolated, excellent examples of good practice. The charity says they urgently need to be scaled up and that the forthcoming NHS Ten Year Plan is well-placed to be the vehicle for driving this through.

The data shows that of older people aged 65:

- 10% (1.1 million) of older people have difficult dressing
- 5% (500,000) of older people have difficulty walking across a room
- 6% (640,000) of older people have difficulty bathing
- 1% (140,000) of older people have difficulty eating
- 6% (600,000) of older people have difficulty getting in and out of bed
- 4% (440,000) of older people have difficulty going to the toilet

Other key findings include:

- The number of people over 75 has grown by 18% since 2017
- Yet fewer older people are receiving local authority long term care (542,420 in 2022/23 compared to 565,240 in 2017/18)
- Growth in the number of GPs is not keeping pace with the population growth of older people aged 75+

The risk of needing to attend A&E increases as we get older: per 100,000 population, there are 49,917 attendances for the 75–79 age group, rising to 93,931 for those aged over 90.

The social care sector is struggling to fill vacancies in almost every key adult social care role.

The numbers of district nurses reduced by 17.5% between 2014 and 2023 – a trend in completely the wrong direction, given how central their role is in treating older people at home for problems like pressure sores, which can develop into serious health problems requiring acute care. Similarly, the NHS workforce is not growing fast enough to meet increasing needs and acuity, but to the extent that it has been growing at all, hospitals, rather than community settings, have generally been the beneficiaries.

The report finds that primary (GP) and community health services, and social care, are either simply inadequate in terms of availability or are insufficiently joined up and planned. The charity says services must work better together in ways that enable older people in declining health to be identified and assessed, and the provision then has to be in place so they can benefit from early intervention and proactive support. Moving to a position where all these things happen, not just in some places, but everywhere, is the big challenge we face and is likely to require a shift of resources out of hospitals and into the community.

Caroline Abrahams, Charity Director at Age UK said: 'It's deeply worrying that the numbers of older people living with some unmet need for social care have now reached 2 million, out of a total older population in England of about 11 million. Some of these older people may be just about managing, but others will undoubtedly be struggling badly with everyday tasks like getting out of bed and washing, increasing their risk of problems like falls which could cause them serious injury, or worse.'

'The Government has not yet said what it intends to do in terms of reforming and refinancing social care, though it has made it clear that it sees social care playing a crucial role in the more joined up, community-based health and care approach it wants to see supporting older people to stay fit and well at home. We completely agree with Ministers and with Lord Darzi that this is the right direction of travel, but the question we would ask is whether it will prove possible to achieve this without the comprehensive social care reform which Ministers suggest it will be impossible to achieve during this Parliament.

'Our fear is that unless this Government grasps the nettle of social care reform firmly and quickly, they will find it impossible to stabilise and strengthen the NHS either, to the enormous detriment of all of us but of older people, its principal client group, most of all.

'Some of the findings in our new report are frightening, in that they show how badly our health and care system is currently failing some older people, the oldest old especially, despite the professionalism and commitment of many kind and dedicated staff. These older people do not have time on their side and it is above all for their sake that we would urge the Government to work with the NHS, local government and charities like Age UK too, to chart a path to a better future for health and equally for social care.'

Age UK recommendations

The NHS

Ensure every Integrated Care System – the body responsible for health and care services in each area – puts in place an Ageing Well Strategy, including how they will invest in public health over the life course and into older age.

Invest in GP practices, primary care and community services to offer coordinated support for people living with long-term conditions and/or frailty. Investment is needed in the workforce, premises and technology.

Introduce an ambitious preventative public health strategy which encourages and enables physical activity among older people and those with long term health conditions, building on Sport England's 'We are Undefeatable' programme.

Significantly expand the number of 'integrated neighbourhood teams' bringing together health and social care professionals with a range of other support workers to help older people with complex needs to maximise their health and independence.

Implement a strategy to clear waiting lists, including a return to the 18-week standard and support for people while they are waiting.

Implement the NHS Workforce Plan, and make sure that all healthcare professionals have the skills they need to support an ageing population.

Social care

Stabilise the social care sector and act quickly to consult on putting funding on a sustainable footing.

Within 18 months, publish a comprehensive plan to reform social care and commit to implementing it during this Parliament.

Fund an immediate pay rise for care professionals, and within two years publish a comprehensive social care workforce plan, joined up with the NHS Workforce Plan.

Introduce a right to at least five days of paid carer's leave, plus a longer period of unpaid leave.

Significantly increase access to respite services and practical support for carers that recognises the specific needs of older carers.

26 September 2024

www.ageuk.org.uk

Social care activity

In small groups, brainstorm some ideas on how social care for elderly people could be improved.

Social care debate

As a class, debate the need for people to have the right to paid carer's leave. Half of the class will support this, and half will oppose.

Navigating Later Life

Chapter 4

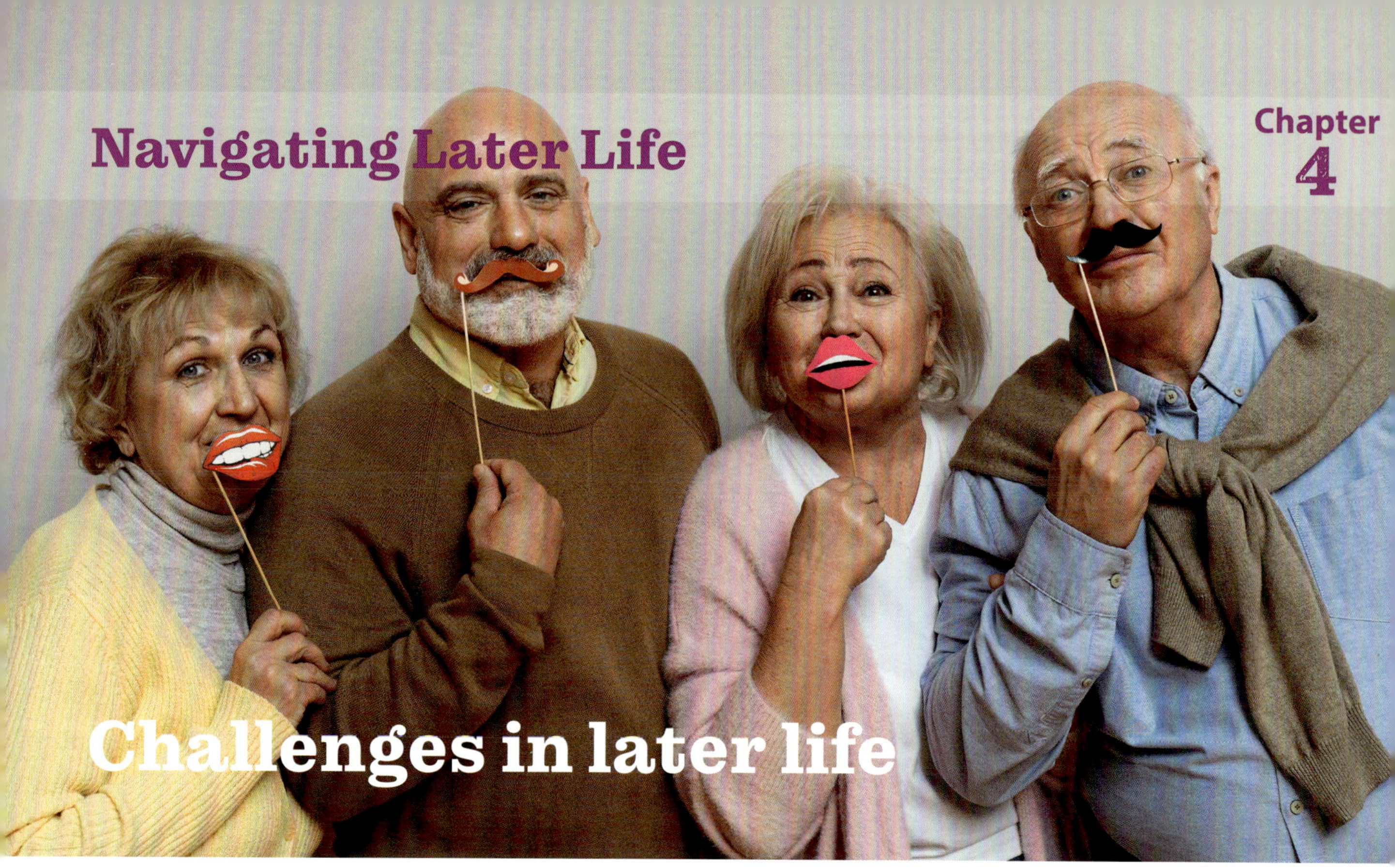

Challenges in later life

The global population is ageing at an unprecedented rate. According to the World Health Organization, by 2030, one in six people in the world will be aged 60 years or over. By 2050, the world's population of people aged 60 years and older will double (2.1 billion).

Advances in healthcare and improvements in living standards have extended life expectancy, resulting in a growing proportion of people aged 65 and over. While this demographic shift presents opportunities – such as the wealth of experience that older adults contribute – it also brings to light a variety of practical challenges and pervasive social stereotypes.

Practical challenges faced by elderly people

Health issues: As people age, they are more likely to experience chronic illnesses such as arthritis, diabetes or heart disease. Mobility may decline due to joint pain or muscle weakness, while sensory functions – notably sight and hearing – can deteriorate, making everyday tasks more difficult.

Financial difficulties: Retirement usually means living on a fixed income. Pensions and savings may struggle to keep pace with inflation, and rising healthcare costs can quickly erode financial security. This situation is exacerbated for those who lack adequate private pensions or have faced gaps in employment.

Social isolation: The loss of friends or family through death or relocation can leave older adults feeling lonely. Mobility restrictions may limit their ability to attend social events, and the rapid shift towards digital communication can exclude those unfamiliar with smartphones or computers.

Access to services: Public transport can be daunting for those with mobility issues, while people living in rural areas may face even longer journeys to medical appointments. Healthcare systems are often stretched, leading to longer waiting times and less personalised care. Social support services, such as day centres or home-help schemes, may be underfunded or difficult to access.

Common stereotypes about elderly people

Portrayal as frail and dependent: Media and popular culture often depict older adults as physically weak and in need of constant care. Such images reinforce the belief that all elderly people lack autonomy.

Assumptions about learning and technology: It is frequently assumed that older individuals cannot master new skills or use modern devices. Phrases such as 'I'm too old for that' become self-fulfilling prophecies when opportunities for digital training are limited.

Resistance to change: A widespread stereotype suggests that elderly people are set in their ways and uninterested in new experiences. This overlooks the many who embrace hobbies, travel and social activism in later life.

Ageism in employment and healthcare: Beliefs about diminished capacity can lead employers to overlook older candidates, regardless of their expertise. In medical contexts, symptoms may be dismissed as 'just ageing', delaying diagnosis and treatment.

Impact of stereotypes on elderly people

Negative stereotypes can significantly affect older adults' wellbeing. When repeatedly exposed to portrayals of frailty, individuals may internalise these views, leading to lower self-esteem and reduced confidence. Opportunities for paid work or volunteering may be limited, further isolating them from community life. In healthcare, professionals who attribute symptoms solely to ageing risk overlooking treatable conditions. The combined effect is an increase in loneliness, anxiety and depression among older populations.

Navigating challenges: the difficulties older people in the UK encounter when accessing services

In the rapidly evolving landscape of service provision, older individuals in the United Kingdom often find themselves facing a myriad of challenges when attempting to access essential services. From healthcare to technology, the difficulties encountered by older people are multifaceted and impact their overall wellbeing. This blog aims to shed light on the various obstacles faced by older people in the UK and advocates for the creation of more inclusive and age-friendly services.

1. Digital exclusion

One of the most significant challenges faced by older individuals is the digital divide. With the increasing digitisation of services, many essential activities have moved online. From banking and shopping to healthcare appointments and social interactions, the digital realm has become integral to modern life. Unfortunately, a considerable portion of the elderly population may lack the necessary digital literacy skills or access to technology, making it difficult for them to navigate and benefit from these online services.

2. Complex and bureaucratic systems

Navigating bureaucratic systems can be daunting for anyone, but for older individuals, it can be particularly challenging. The complex paperwork and processes involved in accessing healthcare, social services, or financial assistance can be overwhelming. The need for clear communication, simplified procedures, and empathetic support is crucial to ensure that older people can access the services they require without unnecessary stress or confusion.

3. Limited mobility and transportation

Physical limitations and reduced mobility can pose significant barriers to accessing services for older individuals. The lack of accessible public transportation, coupled with the challenges of navigating uneven pavements and stairs, makes it difficult for seniors to reach essential destinations such as healthcare facilities, community centres, or even social gatherings. Addressing these infrastructure issues is vital to fostering a more inclusive environment for older people. Combine with the difficulties is accessing appropriate transportation, particularly in rural areas, and the difficulties are amplified.

4. Ageism and stereotyping

Ageism remains a pervasive issue in society, and older individuals often encounter stereotypes that contribute to their marginalisation. These stereotypes can influence how services are designed and delivered, potentially overlooking the diverse needs and capabilities of older people. Creating awareness and promoting age-friendly policies can help combat ageist attitudes and ensure that services are tailored to meet the specific requirements of the older population.

5. Healthcare disparities

Accessing quality healthcare is a fundamental right, yet older individuals in the UK face challenges in this regard. Long waiting times for appointments, limited availability of home care services, and a lack of geriatric specialists contribute to healthcare disparities. A comprehensive approach that considers the unique healthcare needs of older individuals is essential for addressing these disparities and ensuring they receive the care they deserve.

6. Lack of accountability by service providers

Working directly with the public, we all too often encounter the situation where an older person has called an organisation and has been dismissed by the respondent, or even had the phone put down on them. Then a member of our team calls up, gives exactly the same information, but under the auspices of a 'professional' title, and the response our team members get is completely different. Services providers must do better. It's as simple as that.

Conclusion

While the UK has made strides in recognising and addressing the challenges faced by older individuals, there is still much work to be done. Creating a society that is inclusive and supportive of the ageing population requires a concerted effort from policymakers, service providers, and the community at large. By addressing digital exclusion, simplifying bureaucratic processes, improving infrastructure, challenging ageism, and addressing healthcare disparities, we can work towards a more equitable and accessible future for older people in the UK. It is imperative that we prioritise the needs of our ageing population and create a society where every individual, regardless of age, can access services with dignity and ease.

23 Februrary 2024

Ten facts that show why ageism is so harmful

If you don't think that ageism is a serious issue that urgently needs addressing, maybe these facts will make you think again.

Most people think that being ageist is just a bit of fun. But ageist attitudes actually cause significant harm, writes Dr Aideen Young, our Senior Evidence Manager.

Ageism is extremely prevalent in the UK – in fact, a higher proportion of British adults have reported experiencing prejudice based on their age (26%) than on any other characteristic. And a study of the use of language related to older age in web-based newspapers and magazines from 7,000 websites across 20 countries, found the UK to be the most ageist of all.

But at present, the issue is still not taken seriously enough and there is insufficient action being taken to eradicate it from society. Here are ten facts that show why ageism is no laughing matter but a prejudice that can cause serious harm to the individual. Our new report, *What's the harm?* also details the wider societal impact of ageism.

1. Ageism can lead to older people not receiving the healthcare they need

Studies have found that age can have a significant impact on treatment for physical health conditions.

People aged 75 and older with breast and colorectal cancer, osteoarthritis of the knee and gallstones are less likely to receive surgical treatment for their condition than people aged 65 to 75.

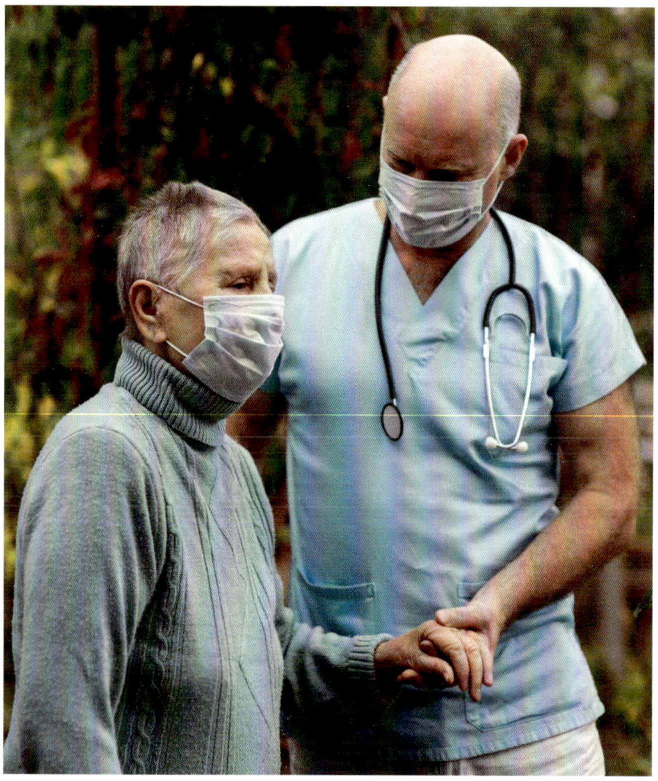

2. This includes mental health treatment

Due to commonly held stereotypes about older people signs of depression and anxiety are often overlooked and assumed to be a result of getting older. As a result, older people with mental health problems are more likely to be prescribed anti-depressants and less likely to be referred for talking therapies compared to younger adults.

3. The ageism we experience from society and others results in us feeling negatively about ourselves and this can be harmful to health

Older individuals who are positive about their own ageing can live 7.5 years longer than those with less positive self perceptions of ageing, even after accounting for age, gender socioeconomic status, loneliness, and functional health.

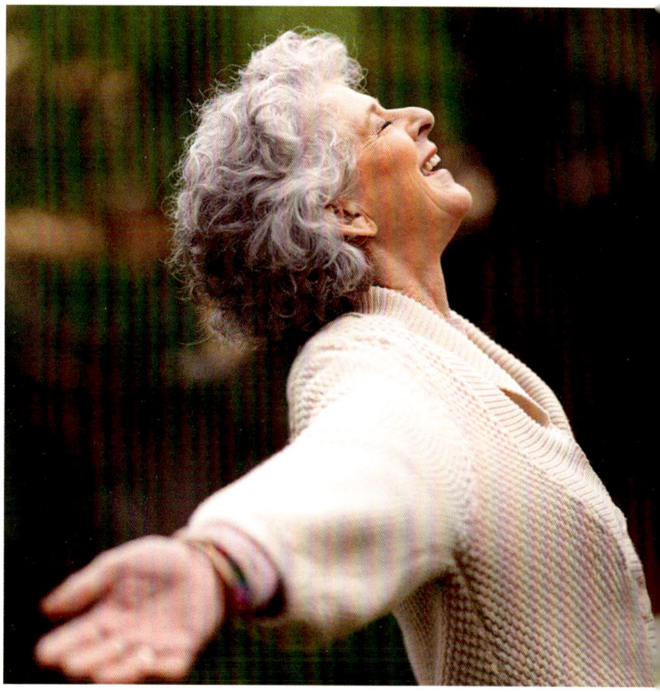

4. Internalising ageist attitudes impacts our own behaviours

People who feel negatively about ageing are more likely to engage in unhealthy behaviours such as smoking and drinking and to have poor eating and exercise habits.

They are even less inclined to engage with health check-ups such as cholesterol tests or prostate exams and to seek medical help for various ailments.

5. Ageism means older people do not see themselves represented in media and advertising

n spite of their large and growing numbers, and the onsiderable spending power that many older people have, hey are under-represented in advertising. Just 29% of TV dvertisements feature characters aged 50 or older. And the ituation is getting worse: representation of older people on creen actually declined during the pandemic (from 34% to 3% with a decline from 16% to 7% in lead roles).

geism can also occur by omission – that is, a tendency to gnore the needs of an ageing population.

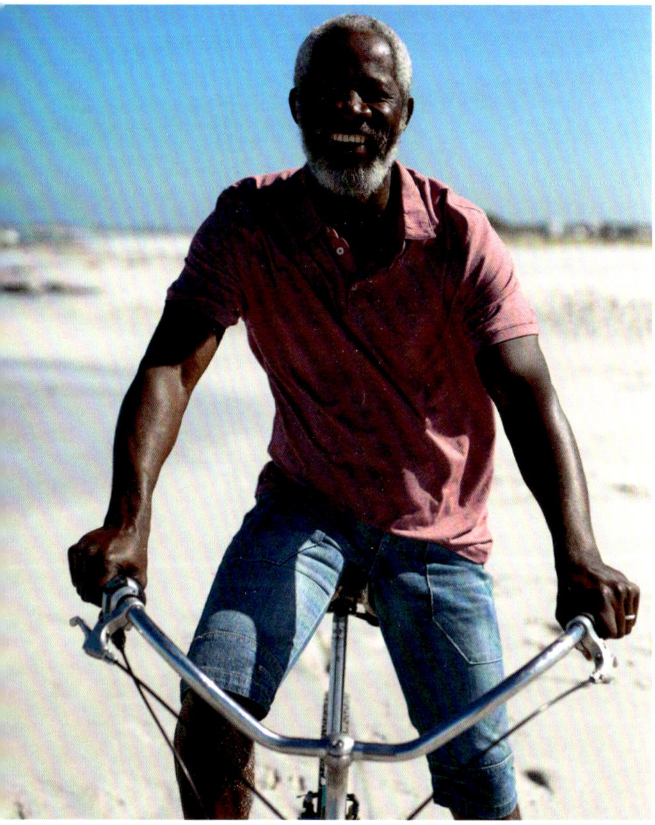

6. Age can be the sole difference between getting a job or remaining out of work

n a study, researchers applied for over 1,200 personal ssistant and bar jobs as both an older and a younger vorker, using CVs that were identical in every way apart rom the date of birth. The 51-year-old applicant was invited o interview less than half as often as the 25-year-old.

Among workers who were made redundant during the andemic, younger workers were twice as likely to be re-mployed than workers aged 50 and over.

7. Older workers are frequently subject to stereotypes.

Contrary to all the evidence, older workers are commonly erceived as being less motivated, harder to train, slower at using technology, resistant to change, lacking the drive to rogress and having less energy.

8. Those stereotypes mean older workers are often treated differently

Managers often believe that it is less cost effective to invest in training older employees so older workers are the least likely to receive on the job training.

9. Businesses that discriminate are harming themselves

Workers who feel discriminated against are less satisfied in their jobs, less committed and more likely to think about leaving their organisation.

Age discrimination – including not providing training to older workers – is not just a barrier to individuals continuing to develop during the latter decades of their careers, it also has the potential to impact productivity and the economy.

10. Homes, but not for all

Ageism can also occur by omission – that is, a tendency to ignore the needs of an ageing population. For example, we see a complete absence of plans to design and build age-friendly homes and communities. Fewer than one in ten homes have basic features that make them accessible for all ages and abilities.

7 February 2023

www.ageing-better.org.uk

Stereotypes about ageing – true or false?

Think

Take one minute to think on your own:

What stereotypes or common ideas have you heard about older people? (e.g., what they look like, what they can or can't do.)

Pair up

Talk to a partner and share your ideas.

Together, make a short list of three to five stereotypes you've both heard.

Discuss

With your partner, answer these questions:

- Do you think these stereotypes are true for all older people? Why or why not?
- Where do you think these ideas come from? (e.g., TV, social media, jokes.)

Get ready to share

Be prepared to share one or two of your points with the class during a short discussion.

Ageism is crippling Britain's economy. We are doomed with no plan to fix it

This bizarre bias serves as a reminder that our backwards society remains obsessed with youth

By Lucy Burton, Employment Editor

Imagine a carer and you'll most likely picture someone young – in their 20s or 30s. Yet there is nothing to say it has to be so.

My grandma's carer Tina threw herself into an emotionally and physically intense job at the age of 83. An enormous support to our family, she's proof that clichés of doddery octogenarians rattling around their homes all day are increasingly outdated.

A vibrant working life is out there for any healthy 70 or 80-something. Now helping a new family after my grandmother's passing, she says the job gives her purpose.

'I am sure I would waste a lot of time if I wasn't doing something that warms my heart and reminds me about how fortunate I am to enjoy good health,' she says.

We could do with more like her.

Sarah Harper, professor of gerontology at Oxford University told the Lords economic affairs committee last week tha the 'number one challenge' facing our rapidly ageing societ is trying to get more adults aged between 50 and 70 int work.

For many working adults in that age bracket (m 70-something dad has no plans to retire any time soon an currently has far more energy than me), the idea that peopl like them could be considered a challenge must soun ridiculous.

In fact, the problem is not a lack of willingness, but reluctance to hire. Many over-50s trying to get back into th workforce face ageism. A 58-year-old told *The Telegraph* las year that she had applied for over 300 roles in 12 month and never got a look in.

One in 10 of the population will be over 75 before 2030

Share of the total population

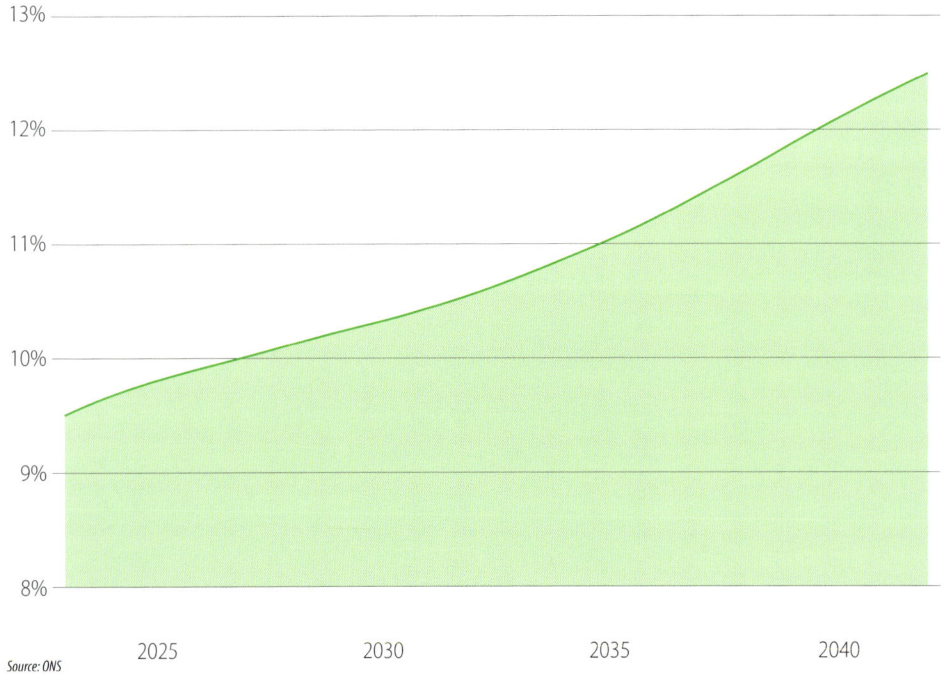

A 62-year-old man who had bee out of work for 18 months said h felt interviews were always ruine by the sight of his 'grey beard'. A 60 year old woman who had worke for top designers said she was ofte told after job interviews, 'We'd lov someone just like you, but younge

Research by Totaljobs last yea found that half of recruiters thin applicants become 'too old' t be considered for a job at just 57 Experiences vary enormously. A report from the Centre for Ageing Better last week revealed that olde workers in England face a postcod lottery when it comes to jobs, wit the South East having three time more 50- to 64-year-old worker than the North East.

That means a million more olde workers in the South East regio delivering an additional annua boost to the local economy wort up to £86 billion.

The idea that workers hit a certain age and suddenly can't hack it needs to be updated. Because let's face it, with increased longevity – official data shows that one in six babies can now expect to live to 100 – the pension age rising and a rapidly ageing society, we all need to work longer.

And isn't there an element of truth in the saying 'you're only as old as you feel'? I thought Tina was in her 60s before finding out her real age for this article.

Emily Andrews, a deputy director at the charity, believes tha if the Government wants to achieve an overall employmen rate of 80%, then it must do more to help over-55s back t the office.

'The Government has set out specific plans to improve th employment rate among the under-25s, but not among th over-55s. It won't meet that target until it does', she said.

he way we think about etirement also needs to hange.

'he idea of a cliff-edge drop ıto unemployment no longer nakes sense as we live and vork for longer. A more suitable attern would be to encourage art-time, flexible work for hose who have hit retirement ge and perhaps want to take a tep back without dropping out f the workforce altogether.

)thers might feel inspired to etrain and go for that career hey've always longed for – one hey feel more passionately bout, but perhaps wrote off in heir younger years as being too nstable with a young family.

 don't think many want to pend their final decades simply vatching daytime TV. With a it of re-framing, this could be n exciting time in someone's areer.

But that won't happen while geist stereotypes still drum hrough society. When I turned n the Robert De Niro movie *'he Intern* a few weeks ago – bout a 70-year-old starting an nternship at a fashion website - I found the whole concept o outdated that I quickly lost nterest.

But this only came out in 2015, and in reality many of he themes about ageism in he workplace still exist today. 'ilms like *The Substance*, a gory orror about a Hollywood tar's anti-ageing quest, serve s a reminder that our society emains obsessed with youth.

t's a bias that feels bizarre vhen so many people I know vho manage staff tell jaw-dropping stories about the entitlement of their youngest workers, tales that could fill a vhole newspaper in a single week.

As Prof Harper told peers last week, getting more older eople into work will involve shifting the attitudes of employers, changing work practices and offering more 'lexible roles. Studies have shown that teams with mixed age groups have better business outcomes.

But more crucially, getting older people into jobs will have a long-lasting social and economic impact that will benefit everyone.

Economically inactive

Aged 16-64

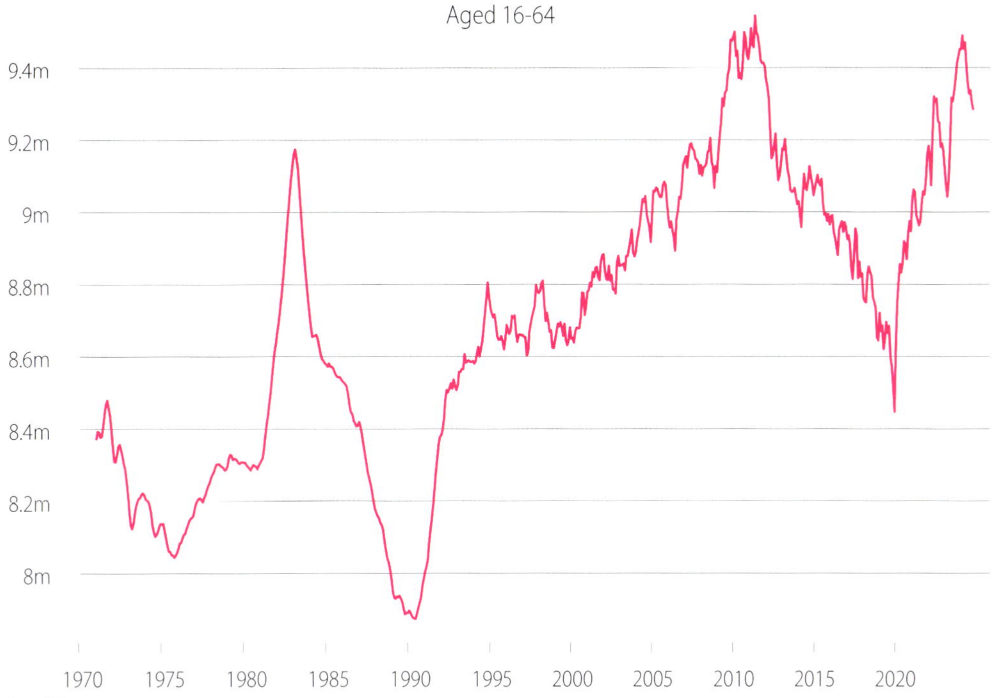

Source: ONS

A growing share of young people are shunning the job market

Economic inactivity rate of 15-to-24s and 25-to-64s, rolling annual average

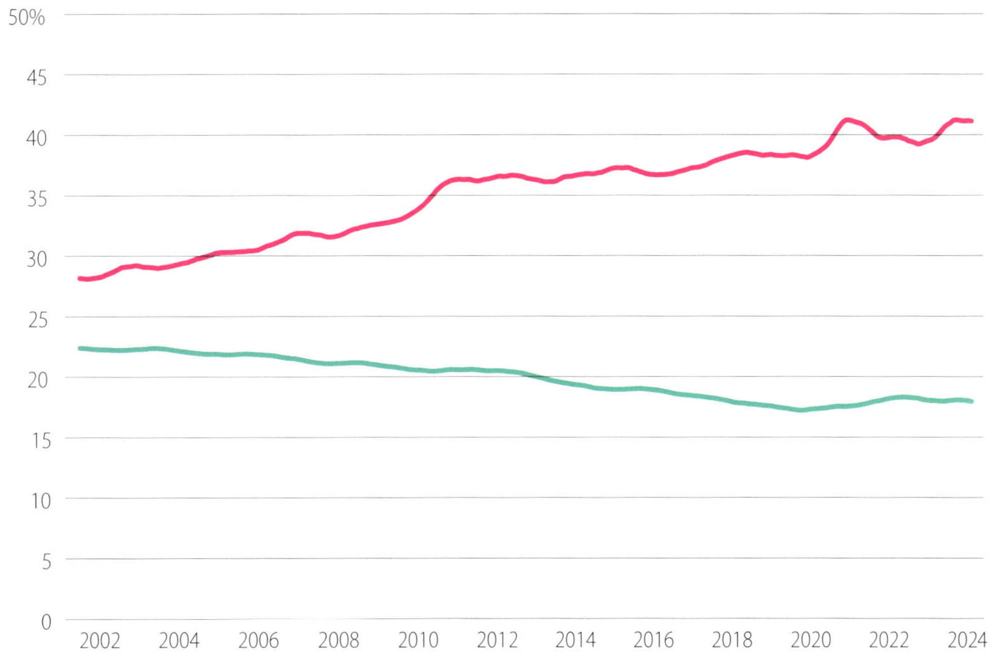

Source: Labour Force Survey

Prof Harper believes that the replacement rate of at least 2.1 children per mother, which the UK needs to sustain its population, is unlikely to ever return. As birth rates plunge to record lows, the number of those aged over 85 is forecast to nearly double to 3.3 million by 2047. Our population is ageing fast. We need more Tinas.

31 March 2025

Widespread money worries for those approaching retirement, new research finds

Almost half (41%) of people aged 50 and over who are not yet fully retired are concerned about living in economic hardship after they stop working, according to new research by the older people's financial hardship charity Independent Age.

According to latest figures, 18% of people aged 60–64 are living in deep poverty. If governments across the nations do not take action, there is significant danger of a pensioner poverty surge over the next few years, warns the charity. The warning comes at a time when poverty in later life is at its highest level since 2007/8, with 2.1 million older people already living in poverty.

The new UK wide polling of over 2,000 people aged 50 and over highlights a severe lack of confidence among those approaching retirement about their financial situation in later life. The biggest concern of those not fully retired was having less disposable income, with 56% highlighting this as a worry. An overwhelming majority (80%) of those over 50 also thought the weekly rate of the full new State Pension, currently £203.85, would not be enough money to cover their essential costs.

Retirement might not even be an option for many approaching later life. Among those polled who are not yet fully retired and who do not plan on fully retiring, 39% said this is because they cannot afford to stop working. Housing costs were another issue, of those polled who are not yet fully retired and renting, a staggering 67% said they were not confident that their retirement income would cover their rent.

The research also revealed a worrying trend, with people conveying a widespread lack of understanding about their finances post-retirement. 48% of respondents said they didn't have much knowledge of what financial options would be available to them once retired, while 16% knew nothing at all. When asked about their general financial situation after retirement, 45% said they didn't know very much and 11% said they knew nothing at all.

Joanna Elson CBE, Chief Executive of Independent Age, said:

'There are far too many older people living in financial hardship, and alarmingly, this new polling indicates that there will be a tidal wave of pensioner poverty without

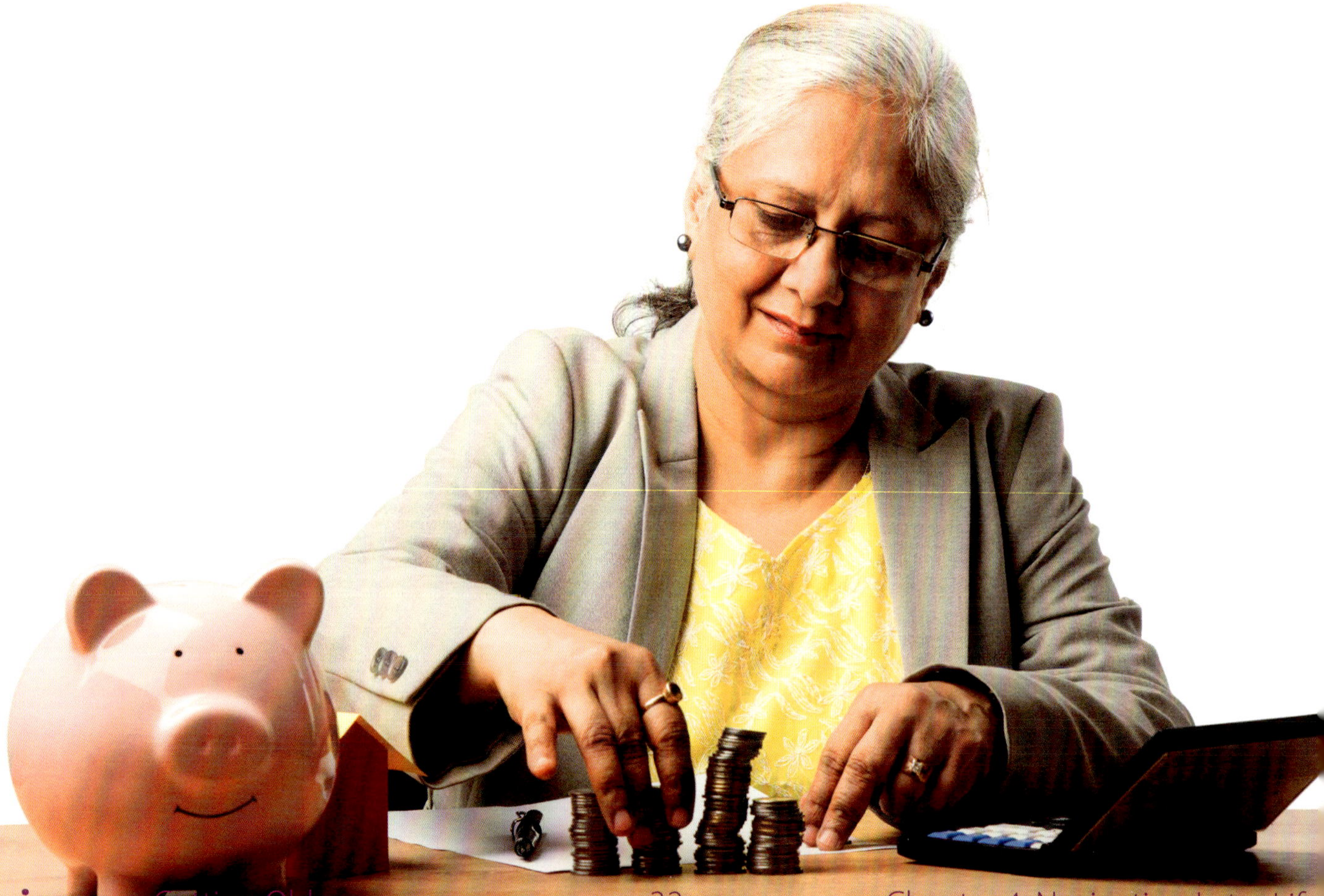

governments across the UK intervening. Nobody should have to experience poverty, it is a tough and isolating way to live, but tragically, it has become commonplace throughout the UK.

Governments across the UK must take notice of the warning signs. There are already 2.1 million older people living in poverty and a further million teetering on the edge. Now we have more evidence that many people approaching retirement are struggling financially and could soon be living in poverty. More needs to be done to ensure everyone receives the financial support they are entitled to so that no one experiences financial insecurity in older age.

It's essential to improve the lives of older people already living in financial hardship and instil confidence in those approaching retirement. Nobody should be left behind in later life, financially insecure and struggling to get by. Everyone deserves the opportunity to live well as they get older.

Recommendations

Independent Age is calling for policy changes that will help alleviate later life poverty in both the short and long term. These include:

- Governments across the nations should increase uptake of social security payments including Pension Credit which currently has an uptake rate of only 63% across Great Britain.
- The UK Government should pass the Renters Reform Bill to protect older people in the rental market.
- National and local government, and utility companies should pro-actively promote social tariffs that reduce costs of essential utilities including water, broadband and energy.
- The UK Government should support a pilot exercise to test an auto-appointment system for the Pension Wise guidance service.
- The UK Government should create an independent commissioner for older people to raise awareness of the issues impacting those in later life.
- The UK Government should initiate a cross-party review to agree what level of income is needed in older age.

Rob, 67, from Cornwall, still works as a taxi driver. He says he has to work as he cannot afford to live on just his State Pension:

'I've had my State Pension for just under a year, but I wouldn't be able to survive on it alone. I have to work. The rent here is £675 per month, the council tax is £104 per month, and the water is paid for, but I have to pay for the electric. I'm frugal – I'll do a batch of cooking and keep the lights off – and when it's cold I rarely turn on the heating. It's just a tiny flat with

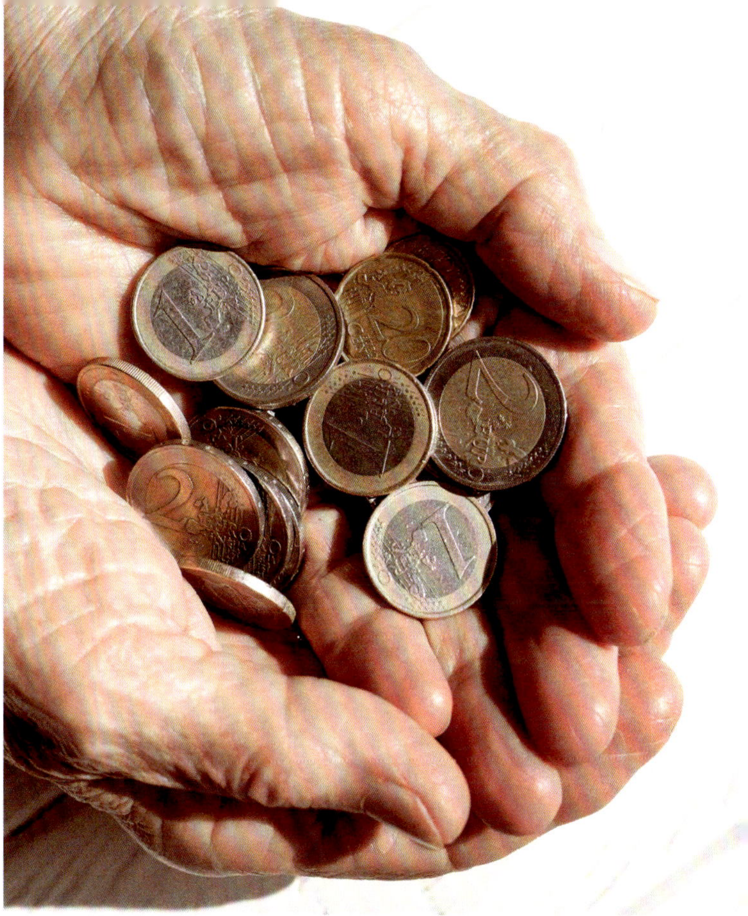

electric storage heaters. I only signed a six-month contract; it will be on a monthly basis after that.

'I'm trying to save money. I'm going vegetarian, I don't drink, but I run a car and have to get dental work done, so any money I accumulate just goes. I never looked at prices before but now I do because I've only got a certain amount of disposable income, and I still have debts to pay off.'

Pension credit

There is financial support available to older people living on a low income. Pension Credit is an entitlement that tops up income to a minimum level, it also opens the door to other benefits including Council Tax reduction, Cold Weather Payments and money towards optical and dental treatment. However, Pension Credit has had a stubbornly low uptake for years. The latest figures for Great Britain showed that only 63% of eligible people were receiving the entitlement, meaning a massive 880,000 could be missing out.

Independent Age is calling on the UK Government to urgently introduce a Pension Credit uptake strategy. This should include details on targeted plans that gets money directly into the pockets of those that need support. Previous research by Independent Age showed that increasing uptake could lift more than 400,000 older people out of income poverty and halve severe income poverty to 4%.

29 February 2024

The radical plan for a futuristic age-friendly neighbourhood in Manchester

£1.5 billion of funding has been granted to transform a hospital into a neighbourhood designed for people to thrive as they age.

By Chris Osuh, Community Affairs Correspondent

Futuristic planning for spaces where people can age well and live in an area designed for them to grow old in is accelerating in the UK with a radical project backed by £1.5 billion of funding.

The plan to transform a hospital into the first neighbourhood in the country designed for people to thrive as they age will be a national testbed for holistic health and social care approaches. It will include hi-tech homes that adapt to occupants' life stage and care needs, transport, a village green and a social calendar to combat isolation.

The master plan for the North Manchester General Hospital (NMGH) redevelopment in the Crumpsall district is the result of collaboration by public health officials, local politicians, experts and architects.

Michelle Humphreys, the director of strategic projects for Manchester University NHS foundation trust (MFT), described it as a neighbourhood that 'adapts around people as they go through life', powered by advances in medical wearables and remote monitoring.

The Government has formally approved up to £1.5 billion funding for NMGH under the new hospitals programme, clearing the way for an outline business case for the neighbourhood. The first phase of land is expected to become available this year.

Bev Craig, the leader of Manchester City Council, said transforming the city into a place where people thrive as they age was a fundamental focus of regeneration.

NMGH's 'healthy neighbourhood' scheme is multigenerational. It will include family housing and will be built in line with age-friendly concepts, spearheaded by the World Health Organization (WHO) in response to two major trends – the ageing population and urbanisation.

By 2050 60% of the global population will live in urban environments and 27% of people will be over the age of 65, the OECD predicts, yet experts say cities are often defined by spatial ageism where environments are not set up for older people.

The age-friendly movement aims to ensure older people can still play a part in civic life. The Elders Council of Newcastle, Northern Ireland's older people's commissioner and Wales' commitment to becoming an age-friendly nation reflect how UK regions and devolved governments have been preparing for demographic change.

The humble bench – improved with armrests, numbered to aid in a medical emergency, or placed strategically for wellbeing and intergenerational conversation – can be transformative, with dozens installed in Manchester, taking inspiration from New York's CityBench initiative.

However, the UK has further to go. Akita, in northern Japan's Tohoku region, where 30% of the population is over 65 has more than 60 heated roads to prevent slips on ice. In Singapore, where one in four are predicted to be over 65 by 2030, the Admiralty 'vertical village' has a central medical tier so older residents, who live in slip-proof homes with alarms alerting neighbours in an emergency, can have surgery without leaving. In Germany in 2007, BMW made 70 changes to its Dingolfing factory to adapt to an older workforce.

In Manchester the NMGH redevelopment is expected to transform the 1870s site into an 'anchor institution' providing training and improving life expectancy with two new hospitals, 200 homes and health-tech businesses. There are also plans to integrate existing residential streets into the healthy neighbourhood, where work is scheduled to begin in 2027.

Prof Stefan White, from Manchester Metropolitan University and Manchester School of Architecture, said the NMGH project would exemplify how to free up hospital space and allow people to 'age in place' with the type of support ordinarily provided in a care home made available to the whole neighbourhood on a flexible basis.

Elaine Unegbu, the chair of the Age Friendly Manchester Older People's Board, has successfully lobbied the Greater Manchester mayor's team for transport adaptations, benches and afternoon matinees. She said the healthy neighbourhood would give residents peace of mind at a time when gentrification 'whitewashed' older urbanites with many forced from their homes by health crises to the detriment of communities.

Manchester, where previous age friendly projects include the Derek Jarman Pocket Park inspired by LGBTQ+ over-50s has been pioneering the movement in the UK since 2008. Last month the city hosted international experts at the Age-Friendly Futures Summit.

Paul McGarry, the head of the Greater Manchester Ageing Hub, said: 'The task is to get a national conversation on ageing. How we plan for pensions and care services, what kind of houses do we need, what kind of communities do we want to live in? How do we tackle ageism? It's the last taboo the last acceptable 'ism'.

18 April 2025

Can a robot help you age better?

An article from The Conversation.

By Daniele Magistro, Associate Professor in Physical Activity and Health, Department of Sport Science, Nottingham Trent University

As more of us live longer, can robots help us maintain healthier, more independent and dignified lives? The robots I've been studying are friendly, helpful machines that can talk, remind, monitor – and even offer a form of companionship for older people.

By 2050, the global population of adults aged 60 and above is projected to surpass 2 billion, posing significant health, social and economic challenges worldwide. As people age, they often experience a gradual decline in both physical and cognitive capabilities, which can threaten their ability to live independently.

Daily tasks such as cooking, managing medications or simply getting up from a chair become more difficult, especially for people with mobility impairments or those living in environments that lack adequate support – such as poor housing, limited access to transport, or underfunded healthcare services.

Supporting older adults to maintain autonomy in daily life should be one of the most pressing goals of modern healthcare systems, particularly as the demand for care increasingly outweighs available resources.

My research at Nottingham Trent University, in collaboration with colleagues at Sheffield Hallam University and Loughborough University, explored how socially assistive robots – often resembling a human or pet – and other monitoring technologies can support older people at home to maintain their independence without needing traditional human care.

In our research, we spoke to older adults from diverse backgrounds, including people with physical disabilities and those on lower incomes. Many were open to the idea of a robot at home, particularly if it could be personalised, affordable and easy to use. They often welcomed the potential for socially assistive robots and home sensors to help them stay active and independent.

Robots can remind us to move around, take medication, or contact a friend. For those with physical impairments, they can assist with tasks that require strength or grip, such as lifting shopping bags or opening jars.

But the picture isn't all rosy. A tool meant to help can backfire if it's too demanding or poorly designed.

In our follow-up study, we looked at how people interact with a robot while completing everyday thinking tasks such as following instructions or solving puzzles. One example is the trail-making test, a tool often used to assess how well someone can pay attention, process information quickly, and switch between different mental tasks. These are all skills we rely on in daily life – whether it's navigating public transport, cooking from a recipe, or managing bills.

We found the robot improved a person's performance and reduced how mentally taxing the task felt, but only up to a point. When the robot gave too much information at once, people became overwhelmed. This highlights a crucial finding: robots must be designed with the user's cognitive abilities and limits in mind.

Our interviewees also raised valid concerns about cost – 'how would we afford this?' – as well as privacy, asking: 'What data is being collected?' Usability was another worry: 'What if it breaks?' or 'what if I don't know how to use it?' Some were uneasy about robots making people more passive, or even replacing important human interaction.

Still, many were open to the idea, especially if the robot could be personalised, affordable and helpful. Our research highlights that older people value these robots more when they offer emotional connection, not just practical support.

Designing for real people

One-size-fits-all technology will not work. An older adult with arthritis and a low income may need something very different from a tech-savvy retiree in good health.

So, successful introduction of this technology depends on co-designing it with older adults, not just for them. This includes everything from ensuring that robots have intuitive interfaces, to making sure they can physically navigate a cramped living room, to ensuring they respect privacy and consent.

There's no doubt that helpful technologies including home robots that offer reminders, support, or companionship will be an important part of how we care for our ageing population in the years to come.

But for them to work, we need more than clever engineering. We need empathy, inclusion and a deeper understanding of what it means to age well. That means listening to older adults, testing technologies in real-life settings, and designing for both mind and body.

Growing older should not mean growing isolated or inactive. If we get it right, a robot might not just help you remember your pills. It might help you keep your independence.

6 June 2025

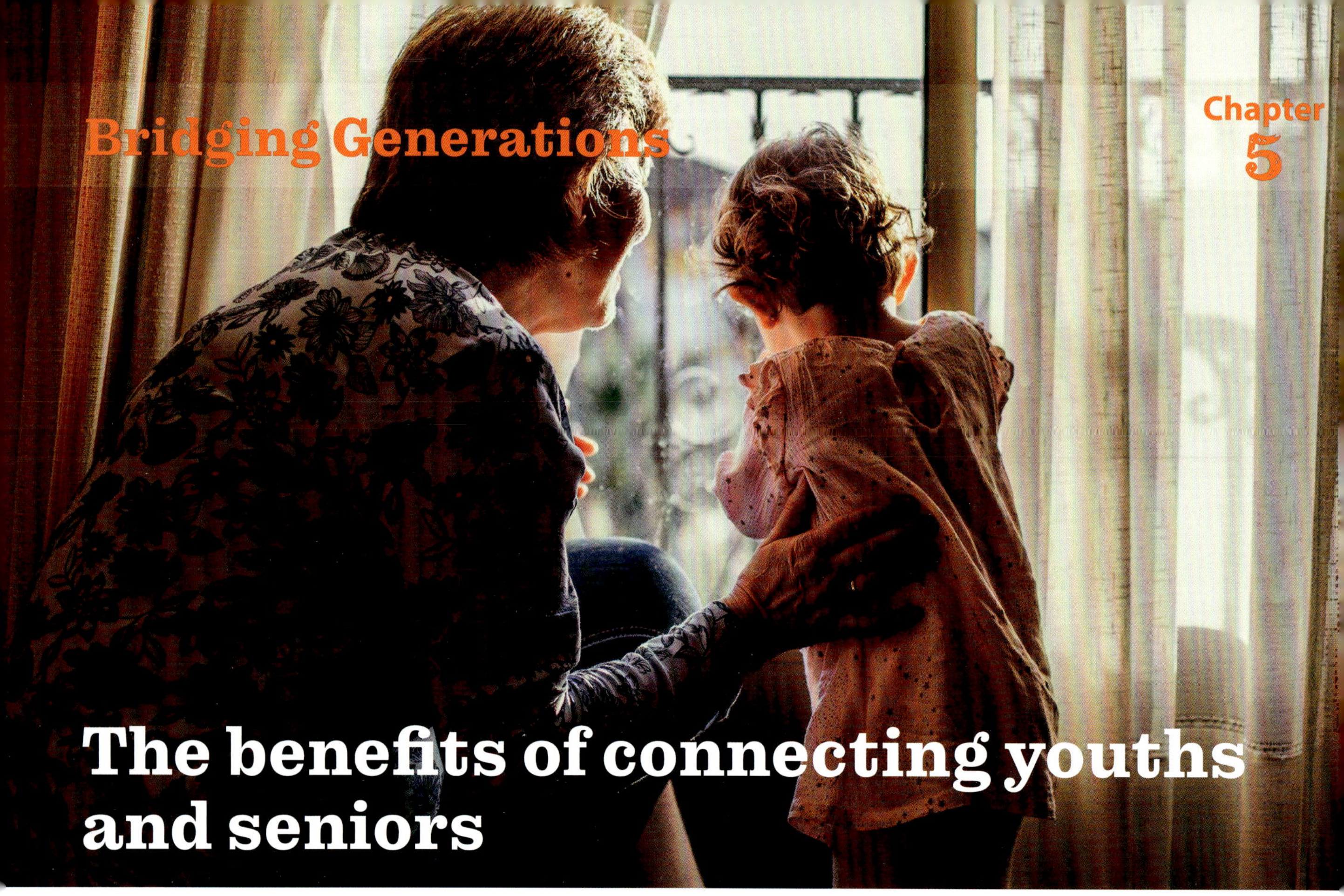

The benefits of connecting youths and seniors

The more time younger and older people spend together, the more both parties benefit. Children have a warm and infectious energy, which can help to bring so much joy to the elderly. In fact, research shows that connecting youths with seniors can help to boost confidence, increase communication, and improve memory.

Children also benefit from intergenerational relationships. Some may not have grandparents of their own and spending time with the elderly amongst the community offers many advantages. Seniors can share their wisdom and help children to develop many of their academic skills. Furthermore, seniors are often very patient and make great listeners. They can give a child their full attention, which any parent or teacher knows isn't always easy to do!

The benefits of connecting youths and seniors include:

An opportunity for both young and old to learn new skills and transfer knowledge

Older generations have accumulated a wealth of knowledge and life experiences that can be passed down to younger generations. Wisdom, skills, and life lessons can be shared through intergenerational relationships, helping younger individuals to gain insights and guidance. Likewise, younger generations can offer new, 'out of the box' thinking and problem-solving to their elders. This transfer of knowledge helps bridge the generation gap and fosters personal growth.

An occasion where both parties can feel motivated and inspired and gain a sense of purpose

Intergenerational relationships have been linked to improved health and wellbeing for both younger and older individuals. For older adults, engaging with younger generations can promote a sense of purpose and motivation, reduce feelings of depression and anxiety, and enhance cognitive function. For children and younger adults, intergenerational connections can provide a sense of belonging, emotional stability, and a positive outlook on life.

A way to share family history and knowledge about the past

It is an opportunity to not only share history and knowledge about your family, but also about poignant happenings within the lifetime of both parties. Younger generations can provide insights into new technologies, cultural trends, and social issues, while older generations can offer historical context, traditional values, and different perspectives. This exchange of knowledge helps break down stereotypes and enhances understanding.

Sharing and passing down knowledge on family history will also help strengthen family bonds and create a sense of unity. Grandparents, for example, play a unique role in the lives of their grandchildren, providing love, support, and a connection to family history. These relationships foster a sense of continuity and identity, passing down traditions, values, and cultural heritage.

A chance for children without grandparents to experience the benefits

Intergenerational relationships provide emotional support and companionship for both younger and older individuals. For younger people, older mentors or role models can offer guidance, understanding, and a sense of security. Older individuals, on the other hand, often benefit from the energy, enthusiasm, and new perspectives that younger generations bring. The companionship and mutual support can help combat feelings of loneliness and isolation.

For children, engaging with older adults can help develop communication skills, empathy, respect, and patience. Older adults, on the other hand, can benefit from the mental stimulation and the opportunity to stay connected with societal changes and trends through interactions with younger generations.

Overall, intergenerational relationships are important for mutual learning and growth, cultural preservation, social cohesion, addressing ageism, emotional support, health and wellbeing, and personal development. By nurturing and valuing these connections, societies can create a more inclusive, harmonious, and supportive environment for people of all ages.

Other benefits include:

- An opportunity for seniors to learn about modern technology
- An opportunity for seniors to exercise both physically and mentally
- A chance to dismiss any negative opinions or fears of the elderly
- A way for children to learn how to care for the elderly
- A new routine which can help to reduce loneliness and depression in the elderly

Intergenerational activities

If you are looking for some inspiration for activities that work well across generations, here are our suggestions of things to try that foster meaningful connections and enjoyable experiences between different age groups:

- **Storytelling** – whether it's swapping life stories or creating new ones, storytelling is a great group or one-on-one activity.

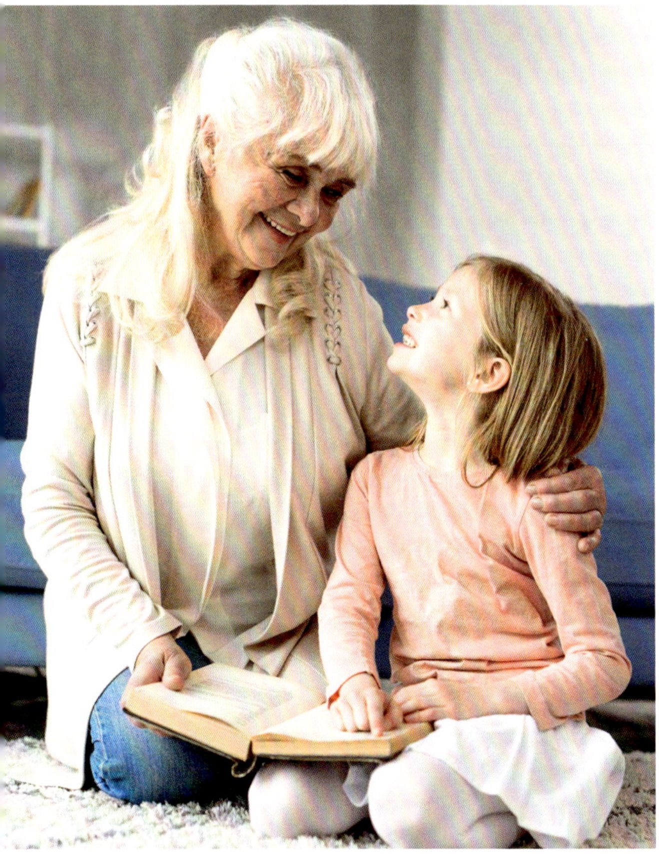

- **Arts and crafts** – engage in painting, pottery, or collage-making to encourage both parties to express their creativity and collaborate on a shared project.
- **Cooking or baking** – preparing meals together is a great bonding exercise as well as an opportunity to learn and share recipes, culinary traditions, and cooking skills.
- **Partake in shared hobbies** – whether you love gardening, reading, photography or music, pair up with a like-minded soul and enjoy together.
- **Outdoor activities** – take part in nature walks or sports activities that encourage individuals of different ages to engage in physical activities together. You'll not only promote fitness and wellbeing, but you'll learn about the natural environment together too.
- **Volunteering** – participating in community projects such as helping at food banks, cleaning up public spaces, or assisting local charities will not only foster a sense of shared purpose but also allows for the exchange of skills and experiences.
- **Family history projects** – learn about your DNA, create your family tree, or simply organise photo albums together to connect over a shared heritage and learn about family roots, traditions and values.

How can you get involved?

A great place to start is by connecting schools and care homes within your local community. Christmas is an ideal time to reach out to the elderly. Perhaps you can encourage your children to make their own Christmas cards and send them to your local care home. This would be a lovely way to brighten someone's spirits and make them feel less lonely or forgotten.

Creating relationships within the local community will bring many benefits to all involved and building connections between young and old is sure to bring many happy memories.

19 February 2025

Brainstorm intergenerational activities

List five activity ideas that can bring children or young people and older adults together – for example, nursery visits, a quiz night, craft workshops or storytelling corner.

Write each as a short phrase and add one note on where it could happen and materials needed.

Consider...

Do you think it is a good idea to connect younger and older people? Consider some benefits to both groups and make a list.

Five impacts Age-friendly Communities are having on older people

The newly published *Age-friendly Communities Impact Report* shows how the UK Network, made up of more than 90 communities and representing more than 4,000 local partners, is having a significant impact on the lives of older people living in their local areas.

By Charlotte Lewis, Senior Programme Manager - Localities

Our Senior Programme Manager for Localities, Charlotte Lewis, explains how all these places are adopting the World Health Organization Age-friendly Communities framework, which encourages organisations in local areas to work together, changing and adapting their local systems in ways that improve outcomes of older people.

An incredible 100% of UK Network members believe their Age-friendly Community (AfC) is having a positive impact on older residents, with five key impacts shining through across the UK Network.

Expanding older people's access to and use of local spaces

AfCs are taking stock of a community's strengths and gaps in the domains of transport and outdoor spaces and buildings. They are finding out how older people experience them, which is prompting changes to the built environment, in turn empowering residents to be more independent.

Many communities have conducted walking audits with older people which have led to improvements to parks, open spaces, town centres, and pedestrian crossing timings and locations.

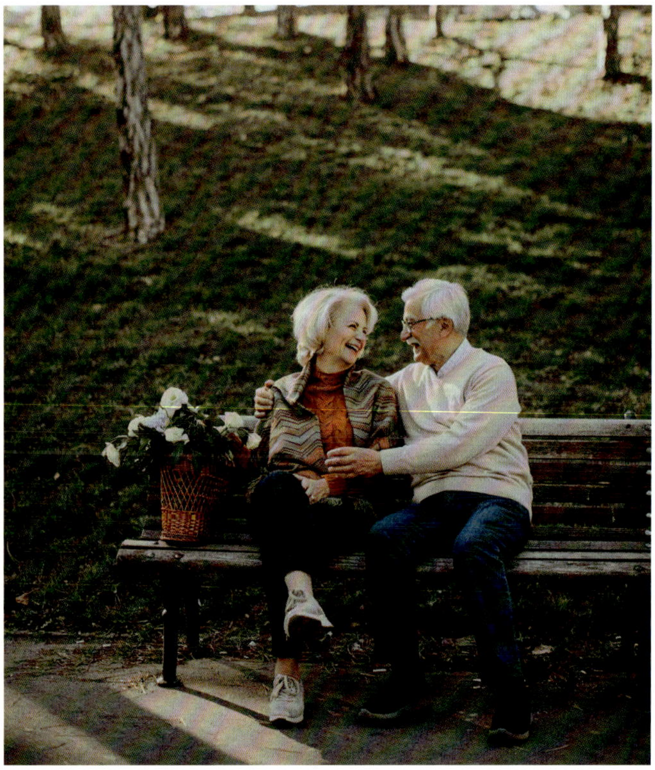

Other AfCs in more rural areas have prioritised developing and supporting community transport schemes. In Barnsley the council worked with older residents to plan the locations for 26 new benches and seats, and Lambeth used age friendly principles to inform their Kerbside Strategy which has widened pavements and added seating and greenery.

Expanding older people's access to support and services

AfCs are improving awareness of and communications around services, making services more age-friendly and developing new offers where there are gaps. Communities are both providing digital support, whilst also ensuring there are offline ways to access services and find out what's happening locally. Others are prioritising financial inclusion such as Newham, where changes to the delivery of their Our Newham Money Service has led to an 80% increase in the number of people aged 50+ supported by financial services.

> 'We have amended how residents can access the Our Newham Money Service, the Volunteering Service, etc. – moving to paper, telephone and drop-in – leading to an increase in the number of older residents being supported.'

Increasing older people's connections to and inclusion in society

Age-friendly Communities run and support many events, activities and initiatives aimed at increasing social connection opportunities. These opportunities connect diverse groups of older people with their peers, as well as creating intergenerational connection. More than 40 Age-friendly Communities celebrated International Day of Older People in 2024, with hundreds of activities including a photography exhibition in Perth and Kinross and a fashion show in Hackney.

Other initiatives have taken a more individualised approach such as Salford's offer of weekly phone calls for people referred to social prescribing. Older resident Diane talked about how this supported her to join her local Tech and Tea session and then to two volunteering roles:

> 'I feel I'm part of the community and able to have a role and worth to society through my volunteering.'

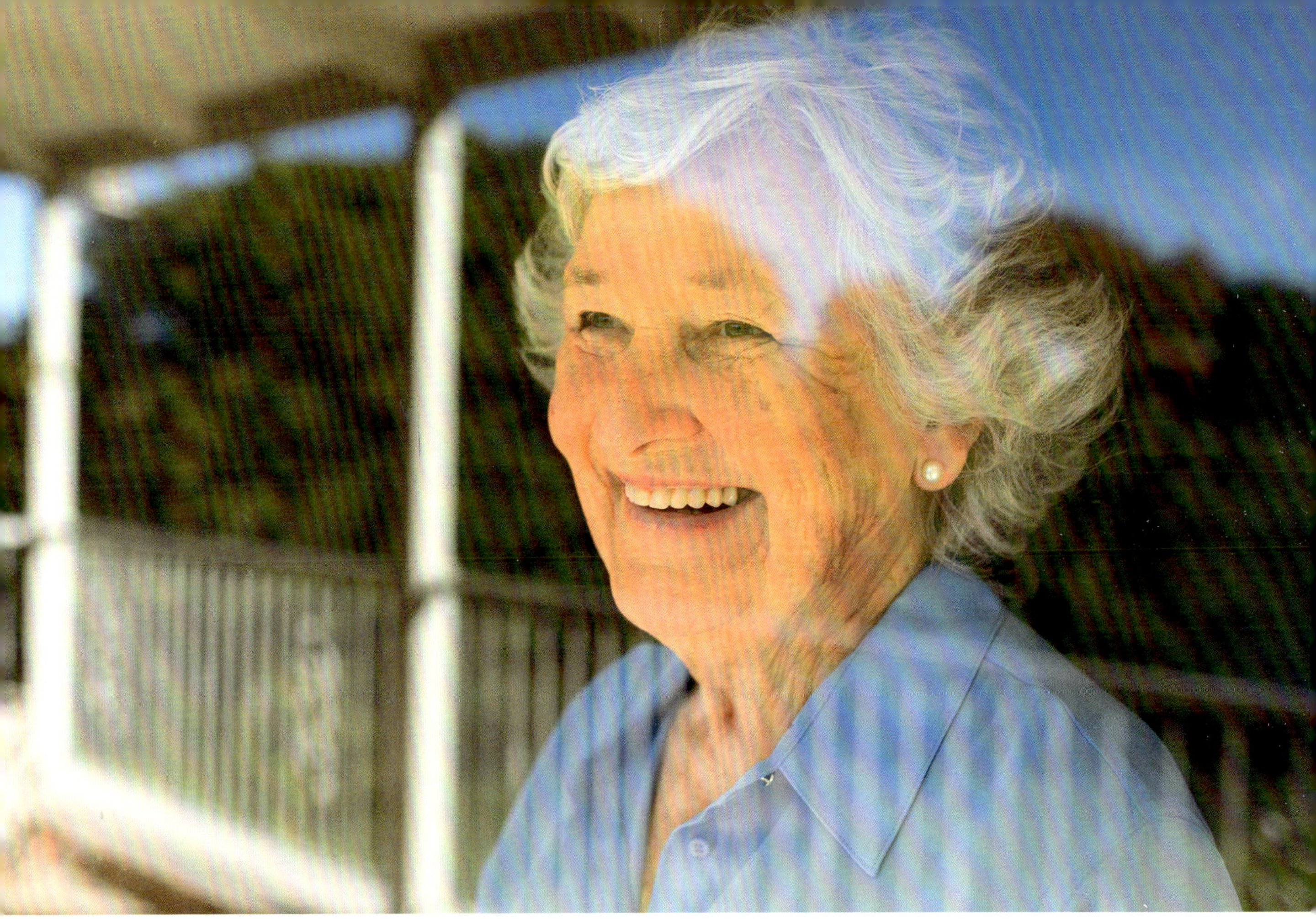

Increased opportunities for older people to have their say in local decision-making

One of the foundational principles of all age-friendly work is ensuring there are meaningful ways for older people to be represented in local decision-making. This can look like democratic engagement activities, such as Greater Manchester's mayoral hustings held by its Older People's Network and Anglesey's Right to Vote campaign where they raised awareness of new voter ID requirements. In other areas they have prioritised developing an ambassador or champion scheme, with almost half of network members developing a scheme. Ambassadors are playing a range of roles locally, from delivering age-friendly training to giving feedback to strategic boards on local plans. Age-friendly Barnet's coordinator shared about the impact their champions are having:

'[Champions] lead our age-friendly drop-ins which take place in shopping centres, health centres, libraries and supermarkets to engage with the public and spread information about age-friendly Barnet. This has…allowed us to better represent the people we serve.'

Improving older people's health and wellbeing

Most members of the UK Network have developed at least one initiative working to improve the health and wellbeing of older residents as part of their Age-friendly Communities. These include strength and balance classes, health MOTs, and nutrition and hydration information programmes. Many activities under the health umbrella are also supporting meaningful social connections, such as Mid Ulster's social walks, and Middlesborough's sensory drop-in clinics for people with sight or hearing loss.

One beneficiary of the activities on offer in Brighton and Hove said:

> 'I really feel it is making a difference taking part in the gentle exercise activities. I can feel better movement in my arms doing it regularly, after a fall last year I'd lost all my confidence, but this is great, I'm making friends and getting fitter in the process.'

More than 29 million people in the UK now live in age-friendly communities and will benefit from these changes now or in the future. The more places that adopt this approach, the more these practices can be scaled and spread across the country. These changes are being enabled across the country through the strength of the World Health Organization's Age-friendly Communities framework and the support offered by the UK Network including capacity building, high-quality resources and the sharing of ideas across the UK.

20 February 2025

Why you must respect your elders

By Klara Coxill

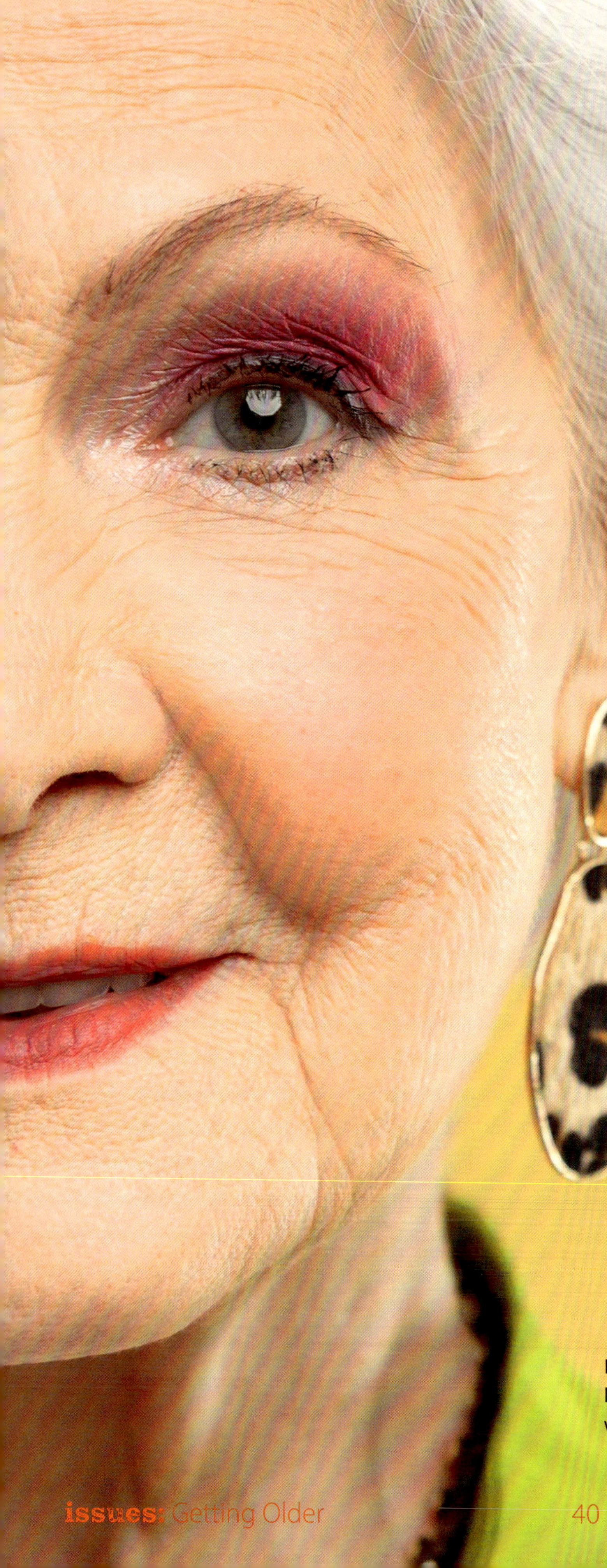

Respect your elders is a phrase often repeated to children and that you are likely to have heard many times yourself. But what does it mean and why is it so important for younger generations to give respect to older people?

In this piece, Lottie delves into the reasons that society should hold its seniors in high esteem, as well as advising on small things that individuals can do to respect seniors.

Older people are often overlooked by society

Despite being a large and growing group in the UK, the elderly are often overlooked. It is common for the views of older people to be dismissed or not considered, with their age being used as reason to do so.

This is ageism – a form of discrimination in which the capabilities of people are assumed to be poor because of their age. Any form of discrimination is wrong and should be fought against.

This means respecting your elders is a vital part of ending prejudice in the UK, so that people of all backgrounds have access to the same rights and opportunities.

To maintain the unity of society

Polarisation has become a much used term in conversations about politics and society. Two groups often pitted against one another are the young and old.

Younger people are told their elders have backwards views, while older folks are told their juniors are naive. Recognising these as stereotypes and reaching out is the way to combat this division.

Taking time to speak with those older than you and enjoy their company can help you to see they aren't so different from you.

With age comes wisdom

Not only may older people share similar concerns about life, they are also likely to have more life experiences and wisdom to share on problems.

Older people's advanced age means they have faced many of life's challenges already and will have useful information to share from their experiences.

Start a meaningful conversation with an older relative or neighbour and you are likely to find they have advice on life worth listening to.

You may learn about other experiences, history and traditions

The ability of senior citizens to teach those younger than them is not limited to life problems.

Years of experience mean older people possess a vast wealth of knowledge to pass on, particularly around history and skills.

Take time to listen to the elderly and you'll often be surprised by the unusual stories that you'll hear about the past. It's a vital part of remembering history and respecting the experience of older generations.

Next time your grandparents start talking about 'back in the day', listen in, they may have some valuable life advice to share!

Sharing experiences between generations aids mental health

Research has proven the benefits of cross-generational interaction, particularly between children and the elderly.

A report from Stanford showed that younger people benefit from strong relationships with their seniors, gaining advice from a group that generally has the experience and time to nurture them.

Meanwhile, older people are nourished by the emotional connection that they form with their juniors. Taking the role of a mentor is rewarding and provides a sense of purpose.

Senior people's needs may be different

Older people may have different capabilities to you and it is important to remember this.

Age sometimes impacts a person's physical abilities, with joint pain or mobility issues becoming more likely as life progresses. This is not a reason to pity or patronise an elderly person but does mean that lending a helping hand is sometimes appropriate.

It may be giving up your seat on the bus or offering to carry someone's shopping. These small gestures can be incredibly meaningful and make a big difference to their day.

Whether the person you help is in need or not, offering your service is a simple and kind way to appreciate the needs of different people.

Elderly people built the society you live in

Finally, you should show deference to your elders because they are the people who built the society you live in.

Just as society must contemplate the failings of history, it should celebrate the accomplishments of older generations. Although the world is not perfect, failing to recognise positive achievements in the past can cause people to feel hopeless about the state of the world.

Listening to and venerating the experiences of elderly relatives or friends will empower you in your own life. Be inspired by the successes of those around you.

Ways to respect your elders

So, how do you show respect to your elders? Simply not being rude is not enough to do this – you must be active in showing your regard for older people.

Easy ways to do this include:

- **Ask your elders for advice** – Not only will you learn a lot, but this will also show that you value their opinion
- **Ask an older person to teach you a skill** – You will get to learn something new, while your relative or friend will feel the reward of passing on their knowledge
- **Offer your seat on public transpor**t – Not all elderly people will require this help, but making the offer is a kind gesture to show consideration
- **Be patient** – If an older person is taking longer to do something or needs a little guidance, remember all the knowledge they have that you don't and give them time
- **Tell older people that you respect them** – The simplest but most often forgotten way to show your regards is to simply tell them

Remember not to patronise your elders

Although showing respect may often mean offering assistance, it is important that you avoid these actions becoming demeaning. You must not automatically assume that an older person is in need of your help and should listen to them if they say they are not.

For example, when offering your seat on a bus or train, you must ask before standing up and should only move if they have agreed they would like to sit down. Continuing to attempt to offer your seat could lead to the other person feeling badgered and even offend them.

24 July 2024

Useful Websites

Useful websites

www.ageing-better.org.uk

www.ageuk.org.uk

www.ariacare.co.uk

www.cam.ac.uk

www.dementiauk.org

www.healthline.com

www.independent.co.uk

www.independentage.org

www.lottie.org

www.ntu.ac.uk

www.opaal.org.uk

www.telegraph.co.uk

www.theconversation.com

www.theguardian.com

www.who.int

Further Reading

Books (fiction and non-fiction

Elizabeth Is Missing by Emma Healey – A mystery seen through the eyes of an elderly woman with dementia who is convinced her friend has disappeared.

The Hundred-Year-Old Man Who Climbed Out of the Window and Disappeared by Jonas Jonasson – A quirky comedy about a centenarian who escapes his care home and ends up in a wild adventure.

The Secret Diary of Hendrik Groen, 83¼ Years Old by Hendrik Groen – A funny and touching diary from a man living in a retirement home, determined not to grow old quietly.

Being Mortal: Illness, Medicine, and What Matters in the End by Atul Gawande – A doctor's perspective on ageing, medicine, and how society treats people in later life.

A Man Called Ove by Fredrik Backman – A grumpy older man finds unexpected friendship and meaning after new neighbours arrive.

The Little Old Lady Who Broke All the Rules by Catharina Ingelman-Sundberg – A group of pensioners rebel against their dull routines by staging a heist

Somebody I Used to Know by Wendy Mitchell – A moving memoir written by a woman living with young-onset dementia.

These Foolish Things by Deborah Moggach – The novel that inspired *The Best Exotic Marigold Hotel*, about a group of British retirees who move to a care home in India and find new adventures.

Films

Up (2009) – An elderly widower ties balloons to his house for a great adventure, only to discover friendship with a young boy along the way.

Cocoon (1985) – A group of elderly people discover a swimming pool with alien powers that restores their youth and vitality.

The Intern (2015) – A 70-year-old widower joins a fashion start-up as an intern, showing that older workers have much to contribute.

On Golden Pond (1981) – A family drama about ageing parents, estranged relationships, and reconciliation by a lakeside summer home.

The Father (2020) – A powerful portrayal of dementia, told through the shifting perspective of a man losing his grip on reality.

Quartet (2012) – Retired opera singers prepare for a gala concert, exploring ageing, friendship, and music.

Driving Miss Daisy (1989) – A long-term friendship grows between an elderly woman and her chauffeur, against a backdrop of social change.

The Best Exotic Marigold Hotel (2011) – A group of British retirees move to India in search of a more affordable and adventurous retirement, finding community and fresh purpose.

TV shows

The Golden Girls – A classic sitcom about four older women living together, filled with wit, warmth, and humour about later life.

Old People's Home for 4 Year Olds (Channel 4) – A heartwarming documentary where pre-schoolers spend time in a care home, transforming the lives of both groups.

Call the Midwife (BBC) – Period drama that often explores ageing, illness, and family bonds through the lives of elderly patients.

Waiting for God (BBC classic) – A sharp sitcom about two residents of a retirement home who refuse to fit old-age stereotypes.

Last Tango in Halifax (BBC) – Romance and family drama about two widowed pensioners who rekindle a childhood love.

Vera (ITV) – A detective series led by a seasoned older woman, proving that age is no barrier to intelligence or leadership.

Our Dementia Choir with Vicky McClure (BBC) – Documentary following a choir of people with dementia, showing the healing power of music.

Nine to Five with Stacey Dooley (BBC Three) – In one series, young people work alongside older employees, exploring differences in work and generational attitudes.

Note: Not all of these titles will be suitable for every age group. Some deal with serious issues like illness, grief, and dementia. It's always best to check with a librarian, teacher, or parent to find the right fit for you.

Glossary

Ageing
As we grow older, our bodies change – skin wrinkles, bones weaken, and memory may fade. This is due to cells wearing out. A healthy lifestyle can delay these effects.

Ageing population
A population where the average age is rising, usually due to longer life expectancy and fewer births. This can affect healthcare, pensions and the workforce.

Ageism
Unfair treatment of someone because of their age. It can affect confidence, job chances, income and quality of life.

Alzheimer's disease
A type of dementia mostly affecting older people. It causes memory loss and confusion. Keeping your brain active and eating well may reduce your risk.

Baby boomer
A person born between 1946 and 1964, during a time when lots of babies were born after World War II.

Carer
Someone who looks after a family member or friend who needs help due to illness, disability or old age – often unpaid.

Centenarian
A person who has reached the age of 100. In the UK, they receive a message from the King.

Cognitive
Relating to how we think, learn, remember and make decisions.

Dementia
A condition that affects memory, mood and communication, mostly in older people. Over 800,000 people in the UK have it, including some under 65.

Discrimination
Treating someone unfairly because they belong to a certain group, such as their age, race, gender or ability.

Elder abuse
When an older person is harmed physically, emotionally, sexually or financially, often by someone meant to care for them.

End-of-life care
Support given to people in the final months or weeks of life, focusing on comfort, dignity and quality of life.

Falls prevention
Actions taken to reduce the risk of falling in older age, like home safety checks or balance exercises.

Frailty
A condition in older people where the body becomes weaker, making them more at risk of illness, falls or injury.

Geriatric
Relating to the health and care of older people.

Grey pound
A term used to describe the spending power of older people, especially in industries like travel, leisure and health.

Intergenerational
Describes relationships or activities that involve people of different age groups, often helping to reduce age gaps and challenge stereotypes.

Life expectancy
The average number of years a person is expected to live, based on factors like healthcare, lifestyle and genetics.

Loneliness
Feeling isolated or alone. You can feel lonely even when surrounded by others if you don't feel truly connected.

Mobility aid
A device that helps people move around, like a walking stick, Zimmer frame or mobility scooter.

Osteoporosis
A condition where bones become weak and break easily, often in older adults. Exercise and a calcium-rich diet can help prevent it.

Pension
Money you receive after retirement, usually from the government or a private fund you or your employer paid into during your working life.

Poverty
Not having enough money or resources to live a life considered normal in your society, including food, housing and activities.

Respite care
Short-term care given to someone so their usual carer can have a break. This might happen at home or in a care facility.

Retirement
When a person stops working, often around the age of 60–70, usually supported by a pension.

Retirement home / Care home
A place where older people live when they need help with daily life, or can no longer live independently.

Social care
Support for those who need help with everyday tasks due to age, illness or disability, such as washing, dressing or getting out and about.

Social isolation
Having little or no contact with others. It can lead to loneliness and affect mental and physical health.

Widow / Widower
A widow is a woman whose husband has died. A widower is a man whose wife has died.

Index